THE ESSENTIAL GUIDE TO AGING WITH GRACE

THE ESSENTIAL GUIDE TO AGING WITH GRACE

HOW TO LIVE A MORE MEANINGFUL LIFE BY EMBRACING LIFE'S TRANSITIONS AND AGING GRACEFULLY

INTENTIONAL LIVING

HANNA BENTSEN

Copyright © 2024 by Hanna Bentsen

All rights reserved. No part of this book may be reproduced, stored in a retrieval system, or transmitted in any form or by any means, electronic, mechanical, photocopying, recording, or otherwise, without the prior written permission of the publisher, Teilingen Press.

The information contained in this book is based on the author's personal experiences and research. While every effort has been made to ensure the accuracy of the information presented, the author and publisher cannot be held responsible for any errors or omissions.

This book is intended for general informational purposes only and is not a substitute for professional medical, legal, or financial advice. If you have specific questions about any medical, legal, or financial matters matters, you should consult with a qualified healthcare professional, attorney, or financial advisor.

Teilingen Press is not affiliated with any product or vendor mentioned in this book. The views expressed in this book are those of the author and do not necessarily reflect the views of Teilingen Press.

To all who stand at the threshold of their golden years, may this book inspire you to embrace every moment with joy, courage, and an open heart.

Aging is not just about adding years to life, but more importantly, adding life to years.

Anyone who keeps the ability to see beauty never grows old.

FRANZ KAFKA

CONTENTS

Embracing the Golden Years   xiii

1. HEALTH AND WELLNESS: THE FOUNDATIONS OF VITALITY   1
   Exercise: Keeping the Body and Mind Active   3
   Mental Health: Cultivating a Resilient Mind   5
   Sleep: The Cornerstone of Recovery   6
   Preventative Care: Staying Ahead of Health Challenges   8
   Chapter Summary   9

2. RELATIONSHIPS AND SOCIAL CONNECTIONS   11
   Friendship in Later Life: The Value of Companionship   13
   Community Engagement: Finding Your Place   14
   Romance After Retirement: Love Knows No Age   16
   Dealing with Loss: Finding Strength in Community   17
   Chapter Summary   19

3. PERSONAL GROWTH AND LIFELONG LEARNING   21
   Intellectual Curiosity: Keeping the Mind Sharp   23
   Creative Expression: The Arts as a Lifeline   24
   Spirituality and Aging: Seeking Meaning   25
   Legacy and Storytelling: Passing on Wisdom   27
   Chapter Summary   28

4. FINANCIAL SECURITY AND PLANNING   31
   Investing in Retirement: Strategies for Stability   33
   Navigating Pensions and Social Security   35
   Estate Planning: Preparing for the Future   36

The Role of Insurance in Protecting Your Legacy 38
Chapter Summary 39

5. THE ART OF ADAPTATION: EMBRACING CHANGE 41
Mental Adaptability: Staying Flexible 43
Home and Environment: Adjusting Your Living Space 44
Technology: Keeping Up with the Times 46
The Power of Routine: Finding Comfort in Consistency 48
Chapter Summary 49

6. SELF-CARE AND INDEPENDENCE 51
Mobility and Accessibility: Tools for Independence 53
Personal Safety: Feeling Secure in Your Environment 54
Managing Medications: A Guide to Responsible Use 55
Asking for Help: Balancing Independence and Support 57
Chapter Summary 58

7. LEISURE AND EXPLORING NEW HORIZONS IN RETIREMENT 61
Hobbies: The Joy of Personal Passions 62
Volunteering: Giving Back with Time and Talent 63
Gardening: The Therapeutic Touch of Nature 65
Games and Recreation: Fun as a Fountain of Youth 66
Chapter Summary 67

8. HEALTH CHALLENGES AND MEDICAL CARE 69
Chronic Conditions: Managing Long-Term Health Issues 71
Mental Health Concerns: Addressing Depression and Anxiety 72
Rehabilitation and Recovery: Bouncing Back from Illness 74
End-of-Life Care: Understanding Your Options 75
Chapter Summary 77

9. THE DIGITAL AGE: STAYING CONNECTED AND
   INFORMED 79
   Social Media: Keeping in Touch with Loved Ones ... 81
   Online Security: Protecting Yourself in the Digital
   World 82
   Smart Devices: Simplifying Daily Tasks 84
   E-Learning: Opportunities for Continued
   Education 85
   Chapter Summary 86

10. AGING IN PLACE: MAKING THE MOST OF
    YOUR HOME 89
    Community Resources and Support Services 90
    In-Home Care: Options for Assistance 91
    Downsizing: Simplifying Your Surroundings 92
    The Emotional Aspects of Aging in Place 94
    Chapter Summary 95

    Closing Thoughts and Reflections 97

    About the Author 105

EMBRACING THE GOLDEN YEARS

As the sun traces its arc from dawn to dusk, so too does the human life cycle extend from the energetic morning of youth through the fullness of midday maturity and gently into the twilight of the golden years. This aging journey is as natural as the changing seasons, an inevitable passage that carries a wealth of experience, wisdom, and a deepened appreciation for life's fleeting beauty.

To age is to have danced with time, felt its rhythm in our bones, and seen its colors etched upon our faces. It is a process that does not ask for our permission; it simply unfolds, day by day. Yet, how we navigate this journey—how we embrace the changes and adapt to the shifting landscapes of our lives—speaks volumes about who we are and what we value.

Aging with grace is not about denying the passage of time or the transformations it brings. Instead, it is about moving through the years with dignity, self-respect, and an unwavering spirit. It is about cultivating resilience and finding joy in the present moment, even as we honor the memories that have shaped us. It is about maintaining our sense of purpose and continuing to contribute to the world around us in meaningful ways.

As we embark on this exploration of aging with grace, we acknowledge the diversity of experiences that come with growing older. Each person's path is unique, marked by individual triumphs and trials, health and vitality, or the need for care and support. But a common thread binds us—a shared humanity that seeks connection, understanding, and the gentle acceptance of ourselves and others as we are, not as we once were.

The following chapters will delve into the myriad aspects of aging with grace. We will explore the attitudes, practices, and lifestyle choices that can help us accept and celebrate our passing years. We will consider how society, culture, and our perceptions influence the way we age.

By approaching aging as a natural, dignified, and immensely valuable stage of life, we open ourselves to the profound lessons it has to offer. We learn to let go of the trivial and to embrace the essential. We discover that while our physical strength may wane, our capacity for love, empathy, and understanding can flourish. In this way, aging becomes not a decline but a culmination—a time to harvest the fruits of a well-lived life and share their sweetness with the world.

What Does Aging with Grace Mean?

To age with grace is to accept the passage of time as an ally, not an enemy. It is a conscious choice to live life with dignity, positivity, and fulfillment, regardless of the years that pass.

Aging with grace is not solely about maintaining physical health or the ability to engage in activities without impediment, although these are important aspects. It's about cultivating an inner resilience that allows us to face the changes and challenges that come with each new chapter of life. It's about the poise and confidence with which we carry our past experiences and the wisdom we have gleaned from them.

This concept transcends the superficial focus on youth and beauty that society often emphasizes and instead honors the depth of character, the strength of spirit, and the continuity of personal growth. To age with grace is to wear your years with pride, not as a burden, but as a badge of honor proclaiming, "I have lived, I have learned, and I continue to grow."

It involves a harmonious balance between accepting the inevitable physical transformations that come with aging and nurturing the mental and emotional aspects of our being. It's about staying connected with others, engaging with the world in meaningful ways, and allowing oneself to adapt elegantly to the ever-evolving dance of life.

At its core, aging with grace is about attitude. It's a mindset that embraces the present while respecting the past and looking forward to the future. It's about living authentically, expressing gratitude for the journey thus far, and maintaining a sense of curiosity and openness to the experiences yet to come.

In this light, aging becomes not a process of diminishment but enrichment. Each year adds layers to our story, offering opportunities to refine our understanding of ourselves and the world around us. It's a chance to share our legacy, impart the lessons we've learned, and touch the lives of others with the gentle hand of earned insight.

As we move forward, let us consider how we can challenge the stereotypes and misconceptions that often cloud the true beauty of aging. By doing so, we empower ourselves and reshape the cultural narrative for generations to follow.

EMBRACING THE GOLDEN YEARS

Challenging Age-Related Stereotypes

Each experience in our lives contributes to the richness of our personal narratives. As we weave our way into the golden years, it's essential to recognize that aging is not merely a biological process but a complex interplay of culture, perception, and individual stories. To age with grace is to understand and challenge the age-related stereotypes that often color our society's views on growing older.

Stereotypes about aging are deeply ingrained in many cultures, painting the later stages of life with broad strokes of decline and diminished value. These stereotypes suggest that age brings an inevitable loss of beauty, vitality, and relevance. However, such ideas fail to acknowledge the diversity of experiences and the potential for growth, wisdom, and continued contribution that can flourish in later years.

Challenging these stereotypes begins with recognizing their presence and the subtle ways they influence our attitudes and behaviors toward aging. It's about questioning the media portrayals that often depict older individuals as out of touch or burdensome and, instead, celebrating the myriad ways they enrich our communities. It's about shifting the narrative from one of loss to one of opportunity and continued evolution.

To confront and dismantle these stereotypes, we must start with self-reflection. How do we perceive our own aging process? Are we adopting these societal views unconsciously, or are we actively defining what aging means to us on our own terms? By cultivating a personal understanding of aging rooted in respect, self-compassion, and an appreciation for the journey, we set the stage for a more inclusive and empowering dialogue about what it means to grow older.

We must also consider the language we use when discussing aging. Words have power, and the terms we choose can either perpetuate stereotypes or help to dismantle them. By using language that emphasizes the positive aspects of aging and the individuality of each person's experience, we contribute to a culture that values and respects older adults.

In our communities, challenging age-related stereotypes means creating spaces that are inclusive and accessible to people of all ages. It means providing opportunities for intergenerational connection, where the wisdom of older adults is not only recognized but sought after. It involves advocating for policies that support older individuals' health, well-being, and engagement, ensuring that they are not marginalized but celebrated as integral members of society.

As we embrace the golden years, we come to understand that aging is a privilege denied to many. By challenging the stereotypes that have long defined what it means to grow older, we open the door to a world where every stage of life is valued and where aging with grace is possible for everyone.

The Importance of Mindset in Aging

As we journey through life, our mindset is the compass that guides our experiences and interpretations of the world around us. This is especially true as we enter the golden years, a period which can be as rich and fulfilling as any other chapter of our lives. How we approach aging can profoundly influence not only our well-being but also how society perceives and values the later stages of life.

Aging with grace is not about denying the passage of time or the changes it brings. Instead, it is about embracing these years with a positive and proactive attitude. It is about recognizing that while our bodies may evolve and our pace may slow, our zest for life and capacity for doesn't need to diminish. Our mindset can be our most powerful ally in this process, transforming how we live daily.

Mindset is more important than you might imagine when it comes to aging. Those who view aging as an opportunity for continued growth and learning tend to lead more satisfying lives. They are more likely to stay active, engage with their communities, and maintain strong relationships with friends and family. This perspective fosters resilience, enabling individuals to adapt to age-related changes gracefully and with dignity.

A positive mindset can also have tangible health benefits. Research suggests that individuals with optimistic outlooks may experience better physical health, including lower rates of chronic disease and a longer lifespan. The mind-body connection is particularly evident in how stress and happiness affect our physiological state. By cultivating a mindset that emphasizes the positives of aging, we have the power to enhance our overall health and vitality.

Maintaining a positive mindset is not always easy. Life can present challenges that test our resolve and shake our confidence. However, the beauty of the human spirit lies in its resilience and capacity for hope. By learning to adapt our mindset, we can approach these challenges not as insurmountable obstacles but as enriching experiences.

In this book, we will explore the various facets of aging with grace, from the practical strategies that can help maintain physical and mental health to the deeper philosophical reflections on the meaning and purpose of this stage of life.

As we move forward, let us hold onto the understanding that our mindset is a choice that we can shape and refine over time. It is a source of empowerment, allowing us to approach the golden years not with trepidation but with anticipation for the opportunities and wisdom they bring. With each passing year, we have the chance to redefine what it means to live fully, contribute meaningfully, and age with undeniable grace.

Overview of the Book's Journey

In this book, we will embark on a deeply personal and universally relevant journey. This book is a tapestry woven with wisdom, practical advice, and heartfelt insights that will illuminate the path to aging with grace.

In the chapters that lie ahead, we will explore the multifaceted aspects of growing older. We will delve into the importance of maintaining physical health, not only as a means of prolonging life but as a way to enhance the quality of every day. We'll discover how regular exercise, a balanced diet, and preventive healthcare can become pillars of a vibrant later life.

But aging with grace is not solely a physical endeavor. Our mental and emotional well-being are equally crucial. We will explore how lifelong learning, creative pursuits, and social connections contribute to a resilient and fulfilled mind. We will address the challenges often accompanying aging, such as loss and loneliness, and offer compassionate strategies for navigating these experiences with dignity and strength.

As we progress, we will also consider the spiritual dimension of aging. Regardless of individual beliefs or religious affiliations, many find that the golden years are a time for reflection, growth, and a deepening sense of purpose. We will share insights on cultivating a sense of inner peace and finding joy in the present moment, even as we honor the past and look to the future.

This book will not shy away from the practicalities of aging. We'll provide guidance on financial planning, healthcare decisions, and the legal considerations that can help ensure your wishes are respected and your legacy is secured. We will discuss how to create a living environment that supports your changing needs, whether adapting to your current home or considering new living arrangements.

Throughout this journey, we will learn that, while each person's path is unique, there are commonalities that bind us in our shared human experience.

This book is an invitation to embrace the golden years with an open heart and a proactive spirit. It is a guide for those who aspire to age with a sense of purpose and triumph. Together, we will discover that the later chapters of life can be among the most rewarding and that aging with grace is not only possible but profoundly enriching.

Chapter Summary

- Aging is a natural and inevitable process that brings experience, wisdom, and a deeper appreciation for life.
- Embracing aging with grace involves dignity, resilience, and finding joy in the present while contributing meaningfully to society.
- Aging with grace transcends superficial societal focuses on youth and beauty, emphasizing character, spirit, and personal growth.
- Challenging age-related stereotypes involves recognizing their influence and promoting a positive, inclusive view of aging.
- A positive mindset towards aging can lead to better physical health, satisfaction, and resilience in facing life's challenges.

- This book will explore attitudes, practices, and lifestyle choices that celebrate aging and challenge societal stereotypes. We'll also cover insights relating to physical health, mental and emotional well-being, spiritual growth, and practical considerations for aging.

1

HEALTH AND WELLNESS: THE FOUNDATIONS OF VITALITY

Our bodies undergo various changes over the years. Nutrition, the fuel that sustains us, becomes increasingly significant as we age. Nutrition powers our vitality and the sustenance that can either support or undermine the grace with which we navigate our later years.

Imagine the body as a vessel on a voyage; to maintain its integrity against the tides of time, it requires a diet rich in nutrients and considerate of its evolving needs. The aging body is a refined instrument that responds best to quality over quantity. It's not just about what we eat but how we nourish the intricate biological systems that have supported us throughout our lives.

As we delve into the essence of nutrition for the aging body, we must acknowledge the importance of balance and moderation. The palette of foods we choose should paint a picture of diversity, incorporating fruits, vegetables, whole grains, lean proteins, and healthy fats. These elements help reduce inflammation, bolster immunity, and enhance cognitive function—critical components to aging with poise.

Antioxidants emerge as the guardians in this nutritional landscape, their presence in colorful fruits and vegetables helping to protect cells from the oxidative stress that can accelerate aging. Omega-3 fatty acids in fish, flaxseeds, and walnuts serve as lubricants for our cardiovascular system, keeping the heart's rhythm steady and strong.

As we age, our bodies may not absorb nutrients as efficiently as they once did, so adjustments may need to be made to our diet. Focusing on nutrient-dense foods that deliver the maximum benefit without excessive calories becomes ever more important. The role of vitamins and minerals—such as calcium and vitamin D for bone health, B vitamins for energy metabolism, and vitamin C for skin elasticity—is paramount.

Hydration holds a place of honor in the body's diet. Water is essential for maintaining cellular health, aiding digestion, and preventing kidney function decline. A simple act of drinking adequate water can have profound effects on well-being.

We must not forget the social and emotional dimensions of eating. Meals are a source of sustenance and a ritual of connection, a time to gather with loved ones to share stories and laughter. The joy derived from these moments can nourish the soul as much as food nourishes the body.

Ultimately, fueling the aging body is about extending and enriching our years and crafting a diet that supports a life of activity, engagement, and fulfillment. With each mindful choice at the table, we are not merely eating but composing the later chapters of our lives with intention and care.

Carry with you the understanding that the foods we choose are the building blocks for a resilient, vibrant body. With this foundation of health and wellness, we are better prepared to embrace the activities that keep both body and mind active, which we will explore in the following pages.

Exercise: Keeping the Body and Mind Active

Our bodies and minds will always seek the nourishment of movement, much like they crave the sustenance of a well-balanced meal. In all its different forms, exercise is an essential component of a vibrant life. It is a fountain of energy that flows within reach, offering vitality to those willing to partake in its benefits.

Staying active is vital to maintaining and improving our health as we age, helping us pursue a long life and enhance the quality of every year we live. Regular exercise bolsters our physical strength, supports cardiovascular health, and helps manage weight. But its benefits extend beyond the physical; it also nurtures the mind, offering clarity and resilience against the stresses of life.

Engaging in physical activity does not require strenuous workouts or gym memberships. It is about finding joy in the movement and integrating it into our daily lives. For some, this may mean taking brisk walks in the park, where the fresh air and the beauty of nature can also soothe the soul. For others, it might involve joining a dance class, where the rhythm of music and the camaraderie of other fellow dancers create a symphony of well-being.

Strength training can also play a vital role, particularly in combating the loss of muscle mass that naturally occurs with age. Resistance exercises, whether with weights or through body-weight movements like yoga or Pilates, can help maintain and build muscle strength. This not only helps you perform everyday tasks but also protects against injury, ensuring that your body remains robust and resilient.

Balance and flexibility exercises are equally important, as they help prevent falls—a common concern as we age. Practices such as tai chi or simple balance exercises at home can significantly improve your stability and agility, fostering confidence in movement.

Exercise also has a positive impact on cognitive health. Studies have shown that regular physical activity can improve memory, attention, and processing speed. It can even contribute to the growth of new brain cells, a process once thought impossible in older adults. By engaging in exercise, we are caring for our bodies and investing in our minds' sharpness and vitality.

As we integrate exercise into our lives, we must listen to our bodies and respect their limits. This is neither a race nor a finish line to cross. Exercise is a personal journey that should be approached with patience and self-compassion. Starting small, achievable sessions and gradually building intensity and duration can lead to a sustainable and enjoyable exercise routine.

In the end, moving our bodies is an act of honoring them. It is a celebration of what they can do, regardless of age. Exercise is a powerful ally in the art of aging with grace, a regular practice that can infuse each moment with energy and purpose. Exercise revitalizes the body and the spirit, setting the stage for a life of vitality and joy.

Mental Health: Cultivating a Resilient Mind

As we get older and accumulate more and more life experiences, we must also focus our attention on our mental health and well-being. Aging with grace is more than a physical endeavor; it is profoundly intertwined with our mental health. Cultivating a resilient mind can help us handle life's ups and downs with calmness and strength.

Resilience is the ability to bounce back from life's stress, adversity, and challenges. It enables us to face our days with composure and recover from setbacks with our spirits intact. As we age, this resilience helps us deal with life's challenges with a sense of intention and happiness.

A rich and active social life can help you build this resilience. The bonds we form with family, friends, and community provide a network of support that can offer comfort and assistance when we need it most. These relationships nourish our need for connection and belonging, which are as fundamental to our well-being as the air we breathe.

Engaging in activities challenging and stimulating the mind is another key to maintaining mental agility. Whether learning a new language, taking up an instrument, or simply indulging in puzzles and games, these pursuits help keep the mind sharp and can even reduce cognitive decline. They offer a sense of accomplishment and progress, reminding us that growth is possible at any age.

Mindfulness and meditation are also powerful tools for mental health. We learn to observe our thoughts and feelings without judgment by anchoring ourselves in the present moment. This practice can reduce stress, enhance emotional regulation, and deepen our understanding of ourselves and our place in the world.

Acknowledging and addressing the emotional challenges that may arise as we age is equally important. Grief, loss, and change are natural parts of life's cycle, and seeking support through therapy or counseling can be an act of courage and self-care. These resources provide a space to process our experiences and emotions, allowing us to move forward with grace and wisdom.

Finally, laughter and happiness are essential ingredients in the recipe of life. Finding humor in life's quirks, enjoying the company of loved ones, and embracing the simple pleasures each day offers are simple activities that can also be immensely healing. These moments of lightness contribute to a more resilient mindset, reminding us that amidst life's ebb and flow, there is always space for happiness and hope.

A resilient mind complements and enhances our overall well-being, and a harmonious balance between body and mind supports a life of vitality and grace. Mental resilience is about enduring and thriving, with every sunrise bringing new opportunities for growth and contentment.

Sleep: The Cornerstone of Recovery

Getting enough sleep is crucial because it helps us heal and stay young at heart. During the calmness of night, our bodies undertake the vital work of rejuvenation, allowing us to greet each new day with renewed energy and vitality.

When we sleep, it's not just our body that heals; our brain and cognitive function also need this time to restore itself. Sleep is intricately linked to memory consolidation, where the experiences and knowledge of the day are processed and stored. As we age, this nightly ritual becomes even more crucial, as it supports cognitive health and helps maintain clarity and quickness of mind.

Understanding the changes in sleep patterns as we age is key to embracing this natural progression with grace. It is not uncommon for older adults to experience changes in their sleep routine, such as taking longer to fall asleep, waking up more frequently during the night, and experiencing a shift toward earlier bed and wake times. These changes are all a normal part of aging and are closely linked to a good night's rest.

Consider how you use your bedroom to foster the best possible sleep environment. This space should be a tranquil haven reserved for sleep and intimacy alone. Removing electronic devices, embracing comfortable bedding, and maintaining a cool, dark, and quiet atmosphere can all contribute to a more conducive sleep setting.

Establishing a consistent sleep routine can signal to your body that it is time to wind down. Gentle rituals before bed, such as a warm bath, reading a book, or practicing relaxation techniques, can ease the transition into sleep. It is also wise to be mindful of diet and exercise; a light evening meal and regular physical activity can promote better sleep, though vigorous exercise should be avoided close to bedtime.

If you find sleeping difficult, approach this challenge patiently and seek guidance when needed. Sometimes, underlying health issues or medications can interfere with sleep, and in such cases, consulting with a healthcare professional can lead to solutions that restore the natural balance of your nocturnal rhythms.

In the symphony of our later years, sleep is the silent interlude that allows our days to be lived with passion and purpose. By honoring the importance of sleep in our daily lives, we not only enhance our physical and mental well-being but also embrace the opportunity to age with the grace and dignity that each of us deserves.

Preventative Care: Staying Ahead of Health Challenges

Another component of aging with grace lies in anticipating and navigating the health challenges you may face over time. It is in this spirit that we explore the concept of preventative care. This proactive approach helps guide us through the uncertainty of potential health concerns.

Taking care of your health early means looking ahead and caring for your body and mind before small health issues become big problems. Preventative care is like a silent guard protecting our health and keeping us strong as we age. This approach to health is not about fearing what might come but recognizing what can be done now to maintain vitality and vigor.

To avoid health challenges, embrace a lifestyle that supports your body's natural defenses. This includes a balanced diet rich in nutrients, which fuel our cells and the building blocks for repair and regeneration. Regular physical activity, tailored to your abilities and interests, keeps the muscles strong and the heart resilient while nurturing the mind with a sense of accomplishment and joy.

Preventative care involves regular health screenings and checkups, which help keep the body in check. These check-ins with healthcare professionals are invaluable because they can detect subtle changes that may signal the need for intervention. Finding health problems early contributes to aging well because it usually means more straightforward and better treatments.

Mental health, too, is an integral part of preventative care. Building a robust social network, engaging in activities that challenge your mind, and seeking moments of reflection and relaxation can all contribute to a resilient attitude. Emotional health is the support that helps us through tough times; taking care of it is just as important as looking after our physical health.

You may also want to consider the role of supplements and

medications. While not a substitute for a healthy lifestyle, they can be powerful when used correctly and under the guidance of healthcare professionals. They can bolster our defenses, correct imbalances, and support the body's intricate biological systems.

Each day is an opportunity to nurture the pillars of our health. Preventative care is an ongoing journey of small, consistent steps—a daily dose of care accumulating into a lifetime of wellness. By staying ahead of health challenges, we proactively avoid the pitfalls of age and elevate the quality of our years, ensuring each chapter of our lives is lived to the best of our ability.

Preventative care turns into a life approach. It understands that even though we can't control time, we can improve how we live through it. Every careful decision we make strengthens how we live our lives, creating a healthy legacy that can motivate future generations.

Chapter Summary

- Nutrition becomes more critical as we age, requiring a balanced diet rich in nutrients, a focus on nutrient-dense foods and proper hydration to support bodily changes.
- Antioxidants and omega-3 fatty acids are essential for reducing inflammation and supporting heart health.
- Social and emotional aspects of eating contribute to overall well-being, making meals a time for connection.
- Regular exercise is essential for maintaining physical strength, cardiovascular health, and cognitive function.
- Social connections and mental stimulation can help foster resilience and improve our well-being as we age.

- Sleep is vital for physical repair and cognitive function, with changes in sleep patterns common as we get older.
- Preventative care, including a healthy lifestyle, regular check-ups, and mental health maintenance, can help you age more gracefully.

2

RELATIONSHIPS AND SOCIAL CONNECTIONS

Our relationships become ever more precious as we continue our journey through life. The bonds with our family grow deeper, and caring for these relationships becomes a vital part of aging beautifully.

Family ties offer a unique form of support and understanding deeply rooted in shared history and love. These bonds are the foundation upon which we can lean when other aspects of our lives shift. As we age, we may find that roles within the family evolve; parents may become care recipients rather than providers, siblings may become peers in the aging process, and children may take on supportive roles that reverse the dynamics of childhood.

Communication is vital in nurturing these familial relationships. Through open and honest dialogue, we can address the changing needs and expectations that come with aging. It is not uncommon for misunderstandings to arise, as the transition into new roles can be challenging for all involved. However, when approached with empathy and patience, these conversations can strengthen familial bonds, creating a resilient support network.

The sharing of memories and the creation of new ones play a significant role in reinforcing family ties. Whether recounting tales of the past or experiencing new adventures together, storytelling helps connect generations. It is a way to pass on wisdom, share laughter, and keep the essence of who we are alive within the hearts of our loved ones.

In addition to emotional support, families often provide practical assistance to one another. This can range from helping with day-to-day tasks to making important health or financial decisions. Navigate these exchanges with respect for each other's autonomy and dignity. Finding a balance between offering help and allowing independence can be delicate, but it is vital for maintaining a sense of self-worth and mutual respect.

Cultivating close family relationships is both a source of comfort and a powerful contributor to our overall well-being. These connections offer a sense of belonging, a cushion against the challenges of aging, and a reminder that we are part of a continuum that stretches both behind and ahead of us.

The love and care we invest in our family relationships are perhaps the most enduring legacy we can leave. Through these bonds, our influence and memories will persist, providing guidance and strength for future generations. Ultimately, the grace with which we age is reflected in the warmth and resilience of the family bonds we nurture.

Friendship in Later Life: The Value of Companionship

As we move through life, friendships become more valuable, adding warmth and color to our older years. The importance of having friends is huge because it's with them that we share joy, support, and a shared view of our changing world.

In our later years, friendships can change and grow. Friends from our younger days might have been with us through life's ups and downs, seeing our struggles and successes. These lasting bonds are rich with shared memories, giving us comfort that we have someone who remembers the past with us.

It is also a time when new friendships can blossom. Retirement communities, senior centers, and various hobby groups provide an opportunity for new connections. These friendships are built on the common ground of shared experiences of aging, the understanding of loss, and the appreciation of every moment. They are less about where we have been and more about where we are now, in this moment, together.

The companionship of friends in later life is a balm for the soul. It can alleviate the lonely experience that sometimes accompanies the quiet of an empty nest or the loss of a lifelong partner. Friends can offer a listening ear, a hand to hold during a doctor's visit, or a shared joke that ignites laughter, proving that happiness does not diminish with age.

These relationships are vital to our well-being. Studies have shown that social connections can profoundly impact our physical health, from lowering blood pressure to reducing the risk of chronic diseases. They also sharpen our minds, as engaging in conversations and social activities keeps our brains active and resilient.

The art of friendship in later life also involves a delicate balance of giving and receiving. It is about being there for others, just as they are there for you, creating a mutual support system. This exchange fosters a sense of purpose and belonging, reminding you that you are never too old to make a difference in someone else's life.

As we appreciate friendship, we must also acknowledge the challenges that can arise. Losing friends over time or because they're far away can be difficult. But the courage to reach out, make new friends, and cherish the memories of friends past keeps the joy of companionship alive.

As we continue to live, remember the simplicity in a cup of tea shared with a friend, the stories exchanged on a park bench, or the silent understanding that passes between two souls who have experienced life's challenges together. These moments of connection truly define the richness of our later years.

Friendship in our later years is an integral part of aging well. It's about the laughter, the memories we share, and the support we give each other that show us we're all part of the human experience, full of life and forever linked.

Community Engagement: Finding Your Place

After exploring the transformative value of companionship, it's important to recognize another type of social connection essential to aging with grace: community engagement.

Finding your place within a community is similar to discovering a garden where you can continue to grow, blossom, and contribute to the vibrant ecosystem of life. Within this garden, you can find a sense of belonging and the opportunity to cultivate new skills, share wisdom, and experience a renewed sense of purpose.

Community engagement is a broad term covering various activities and roles. It can mean volunteering at local organizations, participating in group activities at senior centers, joining clubs or societies that align with your interests, or even leading initiatives that benefit the wider community. The beauty of community involvement is that it offers a platform for individuals to step outside of themselves and connect with others through shared interests.

There are many benefits of such engagement. Socially, it opens doors to new friendships and strengthens existing ones, creating an invaluable support network as we age. Emotionally, it can boost self-esteem and combat feelings of loneliness or isolation. Intellectually, it challenges the mind through organizing events, learning new skills, or simply engaging in stimulating conversations. Physically, it often encourages activity and movement, which are vital to maintaining health and mobility.

Community engagement also provides a sense of continuity and legacy. It allows older adults to pass on their knowledge and experiences to younger generations, fostering intergenerational connections that enrich both the givers and receivers of this exchange. It's a way to remain active, ensuring your life is filled with meaningful stories and impactful lessons.

Finding your place within a community may take time and require some exploration. It's about identifying what resonates with your passions and values. It could be through art, music, education, or environmental stewardship. It might involve mentoring others, advocating for causes close to your heart, or being a consistent presence in a group that shares your interests.

Getting involved in the community doesn't need to be a big task. Small acts of kindness, like checking in on a neighbor or contributing to a communal garden, are just as impactful. Every little bit helps add to the community's strength and your well-being.

As you embrace community engagement, prepare yourself for new kinds of relationships to blossom. The connections made through shared community activities can sometimes lead to unexpected companionship, proving that the heart, like the spirit of community, knows no age.

Finding your place within the community is about creating a space where you can continue to learn, share, and contribute. It's about creating a sense of belonging that extends to being part of the community and the lives of others. It's a journey that reaffirms life's vibrancy at any age and highlights our lasting ability to grow and connect with others.

Romance After Retirement: Love Knows No Age

Your later years, often seen as a period of winding down, can also be a time of new and unexpected beginnings, including romance. The belief that love is only for the young is overthrown with every story of those who have found new partners in their older years.

Love in old age is a testament to the human desire for connection and intimacy. It enables us to experience companionship to combat loneliness and the joy of sharing life's simple pleasures with someone who understands the value of each passing day. For many, romance at this stage is not a whirlwind of passion but rather a gentle breeze that brings warmth and comfort to the soul.

Finding love later in life often means bringing a wealth of experience into a new relationship. It's about understanding that every person has a past and experiences of joys, sorrows, triumphs, and challenges. These experiences can create new relationships grounded in empathy, patience, and mutual respect that may have been harder to come by in younger years.

For those who have lost a lifelong partner, the idea of romance can be accompanied by guilt and hesitation. But remember that the ability to love does not diminish with age or the loss of a loved one. The heart's capacity to love again honors past love and the potential for future love. It's a courageous move, trusting in the chance for happiness and recognizing that life always offers new chapters.

How people have found love has evolved with the times. Social gatherings, community events, and digital dating platforms are now part of the narrative. The internet has opened doors for those who might not have the opportunity to meet potential partners in their day-to-day lives, allowing for connections beyond geographical boundaries. It's a world where a simple message sent at night could turn into a coffee date and the start of a new life together.

In these relationships, the focus often shifts from the external to the internal. Shared values, interests, and dreams for the future become the glue that binds one to another. It's less about what one can provide materially and more about an emotional and spiritual connection.

As we continue to form new connections in later years, it becomes clear that love, in its many forms, remains an integral part of our human experience. Love knows no age and is a force that not only endures but often grows stronger with time. In the next section, we will delve into the delicate subject of loss and how to find solace and support in times of sorrow.

Dealing with Loss: Finding Strength in Community

The connections we make throughout life, from short-lived acquaintances to deep-rooted friendships, form a network that supports us, brings us joy, and gives our days meaning. However, an inevitable part of this journey is the experience of loss. It is a universal truth that we will face the departure of friends, partners, and loved ones as we age. Through our community, we can find the resilience to embrace these changes with grace and courage.

Loss can often cast a shadow over our spirit. The pain of absence can be overwhelming, and the silence left behind by someone who's gone can feel deafening. But it is important to remember that you are not alone in this. The support network around you, both near and far, is a source of incredible strength. Within this circle of care, we can find solace and a path to healing.

When you experience loss, reaching out may feel like the last thing you want to do, but it is often the first step towards healing. Sharing your stories, memories, and grief can open the door to comfort and understanding from others who have experienced similar things. Support groups, formal or informal, provide a space where emotions can be expressed without judgment and where the burden of sorrow can be shared.

Engaging in community activities can be another remedy for an aching heart. Volunteering, joining clubs, or participating in local events can serve as a distraction and a means to forge new connections and find purpose. These activities can reignite a sense of belonging, reminding us that our presence is valued and that our contributions to the world around us are still needed.

In these moments of vulnerability, the true depth of our relationships is often revealed. Friends and family may come forward in ways we never expected, offering support through listening, helping with daily tasks, or simply being present. Sometimes, the quiet companionship of sitting with someone who understands, without the need for words, can provide the greatest comfort.

As we continue to age, it is essential to cultivate and nurture these social connections. When woven together, they are the threads that create a safety net of emotional support. And when one thread breaks, the strength of the others helps hold us together.

In embracing community, we also learn to accept the changing nature of our relationships. New friendships can blossom in the most unexpected places, and these bonds can be just as meaningful and enriching as those we've held for a lifetime. The key is to remain open—to people, experiences, and the possibility that every encounter can bring something valuable into our lives.

Dealing with loss is never easy, but it is a journey that does not have to be walked alone. By finding strength in community, we can face loss and change with hope and the knowledge that, even amid sorrow, we are surrounded by a network of people ready to hold us up. Aging with grace involves recognizing the beauty and resilience that comes from being part of something greater than ourselves—a community that sustains us through all seasons of life.

Chapter Summary

- As we age, nurturing close family relationships becomes increasingly important for emotional support and well-being. Communication, sharing memories, and providing practical assistance are crucial to maintaining strong family ties in later life.
- Friendships in later years are crucial for laughter, support, and understanding and can improve physical health and cognitive function.
- Community engagement through volunteering, joining clubs, and participating in group activities offers social, emotional, intellectual, and physical benefits.
- Finding new roles and purpose within your community as you age is always possible, contributing to a sense of belonging and legacy.
- Romance after retirement is always possible, with shared values and experiences forming the basis of new

relationships. The internet and social gatherings allow people to meet potential partners and pursue new romantic connections later in life.
- Dealing with loss is a part of aging, but strength can be found in community support, new friendships, and continued engagement in social activities.

3

PERSONAL GROWTH AND LIFELONG LEARNING

The concept of time often changes as we age. Far from the frenetic pace of earlier decades, later years can unfold with a gentler, more reflective pace. This period offers the promise of personal enrichment and the opportunity to embrace new challenges with open arms.

Whether learning a new language, picking up a paintbrush for the first time, or delving into the digital world, each new activity we try demonstrates our ability to grow and adapt.

Consider the story of Harriet, who, at the age of seventy-two, decided to turn her lifelong fascination with pottery into a tangible skill. Despite initial trepidation, she joined a local ceramics class. With each session, her hands became more confident in molding the clay, and her sense of accomplishment grew alongside her skill. Harriet's journey allowed her to redefine her own limits and discover a new mode of self-expression.

Embracing new challenges later in life is also a celebration of courage. It takes bravery to step into the unknown, to be a beginner amongst others who might be decades younger. Yet, this act of courage is incredibly empowering. It sends a clear message: age is not a barrier to learning but rather a platform from which to leap into new experiences.

The pursuit of new challenges has a ripple effect that extends beyond personal fulfillment. It can inspire peers and younger generations, showing them that learning and growth are lifelong journeys. Engaging in something new contributes to a more vibrant, intergenerational exchange of ideas and perspectives, enriching your relationships with your community.

When we embrace these new challenges, we experience a subtle yet significant shift in perspective. Success is no longer measured by the mastery of a task but by the bliss found in the pursuit itself. The focus is on the process, the daily incremental improvements, and the pleasure of engaging with something novel and stimulating.

The next step in this journey is to delve into intellectual curiosity and how keeping the mind sharp is integral to aging with grace.

Intellectual Curiosity: Keeping the Mind Sharp

A love for learning keeps us young and reminds us of the unending energy of our spirit. Much like our body's muscles, the mind thrives on engagement, challenge, and nourishment. It is this intellectual curiosity that helps keep our minds sharp and adaptable.

Embracing a lifestyle of learning and exploration is a commitment to ourselves. It recognizes that our capacity for growth and understanding is not finite but an ever-expanding horizon. The beauty of this pursuit lies in its accessibility; learning does not discriminate against age, and the world is full of knowledge waiting to be discovered.

You could turn to books to keep the mind sharp, which offer a universe of wisdom, stories, and ideas. Reading is a sanctuary, a place where you can engage with the thoughts of others, challenge preconceptions, and build new perspectives. It is an exercise that can be both solitary and communal, as book clubs and discussion groups provide a space for shared discovery and camaraderie.

Beyond the pages of books, the digital age has welcomed an era where learning is more available than ever before. Online courses, lectures, and workshops allow you to delve into subjects that excite your interest, from the arts and sciences to history and philosophy. This democratization of knowledge empowers us to take ownership of our intellectual journeys and tailor our learning experiences to our interests.

Intellectual curiosity often leads to the joy of problem-solving and critical thinking. Engaging in puzzles, strategic games, or learning a new language can offer mental stimulation that is both enjoyable and beneficial. These activities keep the neural pathways active, encouraging the brain to form new connections and maintain its plasticity.

In this quest for knowledge, celebrate every new thing you

understand, knowing that each detail you learn and each idea you grasp is a triumph against the dullness that can often come with aging. In these moments of insight, we often find a profound sense of accomplishment and purpose.

A love for learning goes hand in hand with creativity, guiding us to new ways to express ourselves and find satisfaction. The arts welcome us, providing a way to use our curiosity to keep our minds and lives filled with knowledge and creativity.

Creative Expression: The Arts as a Lifeline

Personal growth and learning often go hand in hand in the arts. Creative expression is more than just a hobby; it's an essential connection to our inner being, other people, and the wider world.

The arts offer a unique form of communication that transcends age, language, and culture barriers. Whether through painting, music, writing, or dance, engaging in creative activities can provide a sense of purpose and a channel for expressing hidden emotions. For many, creation is a deeply therapeutic process, allowing them to release feelings and explore new perspectives.

The beauty of the arts lies in their accessibility; you don't need to be a professional artist to reap the benefits. Community centers, local colleges, and other organizations offer classes and workshops for all ages, encouraging you to explore your creativity in a supportive environment.

The arts can also serve as a bridge to connect generations. Grandparents can share stories through written memoirs or oral histories, imparting wisdom and preserving family legacies. Collaborative projects, such as quilting or community theater, foster social connections and a sense of belonging, essential for well-being at any age.

There are also cognitive benefits of engaging with the arts.

Learning to play a musical instrument, for example, can enhance memory, sharpen concentration, and improve hand-eye coordination. Similarly, the visual-spatial skills required for drawing or sculpting can help maintain mental awareness.

But perhaps the most profound impact of the arts is the way they allow for continuous self-discovery. Each brushstroke, note, and word written allows you to explore new facets of your identity. The arts remind us that growth does not cease with age; instead, it becomes a deeper and more thoughtful journey.

The arts become a source of joy and rejuvenation in embracing creative expression. They encourage us to remain curious, play, experiment, and view each day as a canvas awaiting our unique creations. Through the arts, we learn that aging with grace can be done by creating new experiences that enrich our lives and the lives of those around us.

The arts can also prepare our minds for the more profound questions and reflections that come with contemplating life's profound journey.

Spirituality and Aging: Seeking Meaning

As we age, many people look inside themselves for deeper meaning and spiritual satisfaction. This search for spiritual insight isn't just an escape from life's complexities but a deep connection with the core of what it means to be alive.

Spirituality is a connection to something greater than oneself. It can be found through religion, personal belief systems, nature, or the connections we forge with others. Spirituality often becomes more significant as we age, serving as a source of comfort, strength, and guiding light.

The search for meaning in later life is a pursuit that can lead to personal growth. It is about asking the big questions: Who am I?

Why am I here? What legacy will I leave behind? These questions invigorate the spirit, offering a chance for reflection and self-discovery.

For some, spirituality may involve rekindling faith or a newfound interest in religious practices. Places of worship not only provide a sense of community but also opportunities for service and the sharing of life's milestones. For others, spirituality may manifest in meditation, the practice of mindfulness, or the simple act of being present in the moment. These practices can help to still the mind, soothe the soul, and provide clarity amidst life's uncertainties.

Spirituality also can be a source of resilience. It can help individuals cope with loss—whether it be the loss of loved ones, the loss of physical abilities, or the changing dynamics of social circles. It offers a framework to understand and accept these changes, providing a sense of peace and the ability to let go with grace.

In embracing spirituality, we also embrace life as a continuous learning journey. We learn to remain open to new experiences, ideas, and perspectives. This openness can lead to a deeper appreciation for the interconnectedness of all things and the recognition that our lives are part of a larger narrative.

Cultivating spiritual well-being is not about finding definitive answers to life's mysteries. Instead, it is about living in the questions, embracing the unknown, and finding thrill in the search itself. It is about understanding that every moment is precious and that our spirits can continue to soar unbounded by age.

This process of self-discovery leads us to the next contemplation: the importance of legacy and storytelling. Here, we explore how spiritual insights and personal growth gained in our later years can be passed down, enriching the lives of others and ensuring that our stories echo into the future.

Legacy and Storytelling: Passing on Wisdom

Storytelling is as ancient as humanity itself, and the stories we share become the vessels of our wisdom and the legacy we leave behind for future generations.

Storytelling is not simply about recounting events; it is about imparting the lessons we have learned, the values we cherish, and the insights we have gained. It is an enriching way to connect with others and bridge the gap between generations and cultures. As we age gracefully, we become the custodians of our family's history and the guardians of its future.

When we share our stories, we offer a roadmap to those who walk the paths we once tread. We reveal the decisions that shaped our lives, the moments that tested our resolve, and the love that sustained us. Our narratives become a source of comfort and inspiration, encouraging resilience and fostering understanding in those who listen.

The wisdom we pass on is not always found in spectacular tales; often, it is nestled in the simplest of anecdotes. It could be the story of a particular holiday meal that taught us the importance of family or a recollection of a chance encounter that changed our perspective on life. These stories are the gifts we give, timeless and more precious than any material possession.

Storytelling is a reciprocal process. As we share, we also invite others to share with us, creating a dialogue that honors the collective wisdom of our community. This exchange nurtures a sense of belonging and continuity, reinforcing that while we are unique, we are all part of a larger human narrative.

In embracing our role as storytellers, we must also be mindful of how we craft our legacies. It is not enough to speak; strive to speak with intention, hoping our words will empower and uplift. We must be honest yet kind, reflective yet forward-looking. Our stories should not be educational lectures but open offerings encouraging others to reflect, dream, and grow.

As you consider the stories you wish to pass on, consider how you share them. In an age where technology allows for our voices to be heard far and wide, we can leave a lasting imprint on those immediately around us and the world at large. Whether through written memoirs, recorded interviews, or casual conversations around the dinner table, our stories have the power to transcend time and space.

The wisdom we share through our stories guides the young and reassures the old that their journey has meaning. As we age gracefully, take comfort in knowing that we continue contributing to the world's dialogue long after our final bow through our stories.

Chapter Summary

- Embracing new challenges shows our commitment to personal growth and our lasting ability to learn and adjust.
- Pursuing new endeavors, such as learning new skills or hobbies, is empowering and demonstrates that age is not a barrier to learning.
- Engaging in lifelong learning inspires others, enriches communities, and focuses on the joy of the pursuit rather than just mastery.
- Intellectual curiosity keeps the mind sharp and can help us age gracefully.
- Creative expression through the arts offers therapeutic benefits, cognitive enhancement, and opportunities for self-discovery and intergenerational connection.

- Spirituality may gain importance later in life, providing comfort, strength, and a means to seek deeper meaning and cope with life's changes.
- Storytelling is a powerful tool for passing on wisdom and connecting generations with personal narratives, offering comfort and inspiration.
- Legacy is crafted through intentional storytelling, with technology allowing for a broader impact and ensuring that personal stories and wisdom echo into the future.

4

FINANCIAL SECURITY AND PLANNING

M anaging money can feel more challenging as we enter our later years, with income and costs changing unexpectedly. During this time, budgeting becomes a practical skill and a way to create a secure and peaceful life after retirement.

Budgeting, in its essence, is about balance. It balances our resources and the life we want to lead. As we age, this balance must be struck with an awareness of the changing rhythms of life. The budget that served us well in our earlier years may no longer fit the quieter, perhaps slower, tempo of our golden years.

First, take a compassionate and realistic look at your income sources. These may include social security, pensions, retirement accounts, investments, and part-time work. Understanding your income flow allows you to plan your activities and spending accordingly.

Next, consider your expenses. Some costs may decrease as you age, such as work-related expenses or mortgage payments if your home is paid off. However, other costs, like healthcare and long-term care, can rise, sometimes unexpectedly. It's important to budget for what you know and set aside funds for unforeseen events that may try to unsettle your financial plan.

One of the most empathetic steps you can take is to ensure that your budget includes room for the things that bring joy and fulfillment. Whether it's a hobby, travel, or contributions to things that are important to you, these are the expenditures that breathe life into your years and should not be neglected.

In managing your budget, spreadsheets or budgeting software can be invaluable tools. They allow you to visualize your financial landscape, track your spending, and adjust as needed. Remember, a budget is not set in stone; it is a living document that should evolve as your needs and circumstances change.

As you refine your budget, consider the legacy you wish to leave. This may involve estate planning, gifting to loved ones, or charity donations. These decisions, too, should be incorporated into your financial plan, ensuring that your values extend beyond your own journey.

Budgeting for later life goes beyond just tracking numbers; it's about shaping your life's story so that your finances support the life you want to lead. It's navigating life's changes gracefully, planning wisely for tough times, and having the courage to enjoy the good times.

As you work through the practicalities of budgeting, you might start considering the next chapter of your financial journey—investing in retirement. Here, the goal changes from keeping daily peace to staying stable despite economic shifts. With a well-considered budget, you can explore strategies to help ensure your financial security so you can age with the grace and freedom you deserve.

Investing in Retirement: Strategies for Stability

As we enter retirement, financial planning gets more complex. Investing at this stage isn't about getting rich but about creating a steady flow of income that supports a happy and satisfying life.

Investing during retirement is significantly different from the growth-focused strategies of earlier years. It's a time when the focus shifts from wealth accumulation to wealth preservation and income generation. Your strategies must be tailored to your circumstances, including your health, life expectancy, and the legacy you wish to leave behind.

One of the cornerstones of a stable retirement investment strategy is diversification. Diversification is the financial equivalent of not putting all your eggs in one basket. It involves spreading investments across various asset classes, such as stocks, bonds, real estate, and possibly annuities, to mitigate risk. While stocks may offer growth potential and combat inflation over the long term, bonds can provide a more stable and predictable income. Real estate investments can offer both income through rental yields and potential appreciation in value. On the other hand, annuities can offer a guaranteed income for life, which can be a comforting thought for many retirees.

Another strategy to consider is the careful use of the bucket approach. This involves dividing your investments into "buckets" based on when you will need to access the funds. The first bucket, for instance, could contain cash and cash equivalents for immediate needs. The second bucket might include short-term fixed-income investments you'll need in the next few years. The third bucket, aimed at the long-term, could be more growth-oriented, containing stocks and real estate investments you won't need to touch for several years. This approach ensures that you have funds available when needed while still allowing for growth potential.

The concept of asset allocation also remains critical during retirement. It's about finding the right balance between different types of investments to align with your risk tolerance and time horizon. Our risk tolerance typically decreases as we age, and our investment horizon shortens. Therefore, a shift towards more conservative investments may be needed. However, with increasing life expectancies, it's also important to maintain some growth-oriented investments to ensure our assets last as long as we do.

It's also essential to be mindful of the impact of inflation on fixed incomes. Even at low rates, inflation can significantly erode purchasing power over time. Investments that have the potential to outpace inflation, such as certain stocks or real estate, can be important components of your portfolio as you grow older.

Tax efficiency is another concept to be aware of in retirement. Understanding which accounts to withdraw from first and how to organize your assets for maximum efficiency can substantially affect how long your savings last. Investing strategies like focusing on long-term capital gains and qualified dividends can help stretch your retirement dollars.

Take time to review and adjust your investment strategy regularly. Life changes, market conditions shift, and personal needs evolve. An annual review of your financial plan with a trusted advisor can ensure that your investment strategy continues to align with your current situation and goals.

Investing in retirement is not about chasing returns but creating a harmonious balance, supporting your lifestyle, and bringing peace of mind. It's about ensuring that your financial resources align with your life and the legacy you wish to create. With careful planning and thoughtful strategy, you can navigate the financial currents of retirement with confidence and grace.

Navigating Pensions and Social Security

Our financial situation shifts in significant ways as we age. We move from earning money to depending on what we've saved and planned for, like pensions and Social Security. Managing these funds isn't just for financial stability; it's a way to respect our work and the life we've created.

Pensions, once the foundation of retirement security, have become less common in the private sector. Yet, they remain a significant source of income for many retirees. If you are fortunate to have a pension, it's essential to comprehend the different payout options available to you. Some pensions offer a lump-sum payment, while others provide a guaranteed monthly benefit. Each choice impacts your financial longevity differently and can affect your loved ones after you're gone. It's a decision that requires careful consideration, and often, the counsel of a financial advisor can help illuminate the path that best aligns with your circumstances and goals.

Social Security, a program that has been a safety net for countless Americans, is a more universal aspect of retirement planning. Deciding when to start taking Social Security benefits is a pivotal choice that requires a thoughtful strategy. The decision of when to claim should be made with an eye on your health, financial needs, and employment status, among other factors.

If you're married, divorced, or widowed, additional considerations must be considered. Spousal benefits, survivor benefits, and the implications of marriage duration on your entitlements can all influence your Social Security strategy. These rules can be complex, and navigating them is often akin to learning a new language late in life. Yet, understanding them is crucial to maximizing the benefits you've earned.

In managing pensions and Social Security, it's essential to consider how these income streams interact with your overall retirement plan. They can impact your tax situation, how you draw down other retirement savings, and even your healthcare choices. It's a delicate balancing act that benefits from ongoing review as policies and personal circumstances evolve.

Estate Planning: Preparing for the Future

As we grow older, our lives become filled with memories and experiences, and we start to think about the legacy we want to leave. Estate planning is crucial to financial security, and a deep act of love for our family and the things we care about. Careful planning for the future ensures our wishes are respected, and our loved ones are cared for.

Estate planning can be a delicate journey because it requires us to confront our mortality with courage and clarity. It is a process that involves organizing our financial affairs and making decisions that will have lasting impacts. To begin, one must take stock of all assets, including property, investments, and personal possessions of sentimental value. This comprehensive inventory is the foundation upon which your estate plan is built.

A will is often the most important part of an estate plan. It is a legal document that outlines your desires about distributing your assets and caring for any minor children. Without a will, these decisions typically fall to the state, which may not align with your wishes. Therefore, drafting a will with the assistance of a legal professional is an essential step.

In addition to a will, there are other instruments and strategies to consider. Trusts can be established to manage your assets according to your directives, potentially offering tax benefits and protection from legal challenges. Powers of attorney and healthcare directives are also vital, as they designate individuals to make financial and medical decisions on your behalf if you cannot do so.

It is also important to consider the potential impact of taxes on your estate. Thoughtful planning can help minimize the tax burden on those you leave behind, preserving more of your legacy for their benefit. Charitable giving can be part of this strategy, allowing you to support the causes that are important to you while also providing tax advantages.

Estate planning is not a one-time task but an evolving process. Life's changes—such as marriage, divorce, the birth of a child, or the acquisition of significant assets—may require you to update your plan. Regular reviews with your attorney and financial advisor can help ensure your estate plan continues to reflect your current circumstances and wishes.

So far, we have explored the practical steps of estate planning, but let's not forget the emotional and relational aspects. Communicating with your loved ones about your plans can prevent misunderstandings and ensure clear intentions. It can also provide an opportunity for meaningful conversations about values, memories, and the hopes you have for your family's future.

Estate planning is an act of foresight and compassion. It is a way to honor your life and express your love and care for those you will one day leave behind. By preparing for the future, you can offer your loved ones the gift of security and peace of mind, knowing that your legacy will be preserved according to your deepest wishes.

The Role of Insurance in Protecting Your Legacy

The idea of legacy becomes more prominent and meaningful during our later years. It becomes more about the impact we make and the safety we ensure for our loved ones rather than the money we've gathered. Insurance is crucial in financial security and planning, tied to our wish to safeguard and continue our legacy for those who come after us.

Insurance acts as a protection against unexpected events. It shows we've planned carefully to ensure our loved ones won't face financial trouble when we're gone. Life insurance is especially important in this protective plan.

Think of life insurance as a quiet vow, a pledge that lasts even after we're gone. It's a promise that if our passing could shake our family's financial security, they will have a safety net. The money from a life insurance policy can help maintain stability during tough times, helping to pay off debts, cover everyday costs, and support dreams like education or buying a home.

However, the role of insurance in protecting your legacy extends beyond life insurance. Long-term care insurance, for example, addresses the reality that with age comes the potential need for assistance with daily living activities. This type of insurance can alleviate the financial strain of long-term care, preserving your estate's assets and ensuring that the wealth you intended to pass on remains intact.

Similarly, disability insurance plays a pivotal role for those still in their working years. It's a hedge against the possibility that an illness or injury could interrupt your ability to earn an income.

This type of insurance similarly helps maintain your standard of living. It safeguards your savings, allowing you to continue contributing to your legacy without the added stress of financial hardship.

Property and casualty insurance protects the tangible assets you've worked hard to acquire. Homeowners insurance, auto insurance, and umbrella policies protect against the financial repercussions of accidents, natural disasters, and unforeseen events that could otherwise deplete your estate.

Each insurance policy should be a strategic piece of your broader legacy plan. It's about ensuring that the values you've lived by—responsibility, protection, and care—are upheld even when you're no longer there to champion them yourself.

Insurance is about protecting your family from the financial unknowns of life and death. When considering the legacy you want to leave, consider how insurance can be a reliable support in your journey to age with grace and dignity, ensuring you leave behind a legacy of lasting stability and peace of mind, not a burden.

Chapter Summary

- Budgeting in later years is crucial for balancing income and expenses, and one must adapt their financial plans to the slower pace of retirement.
- Income sources like social security, pensions, and investments must be understood, and expenses, including rising healthcare costs, should be carefully considered.
- Budgeting for joy and fulfillment through hobbies, travel, or donations is essential, using tools like spreadsheets or software for tracking.

- Estate planning and considering the legacy you wish to leave should be part of financial planning.
- Retirement investment strategies should focus on stability and income generation, with diversification across asset classes.
- Regularly reviewing and adjusting investment strategies is essential to align with life changes and market conditions.
- Understanding pensions and Social Security benefits is important in retirement, including when to claim benefits and how they affect overall financial planning.
- Estate planning involves creating a will, setting up trusts, and ensuring one's wishes are honored, with regular updates as circumstances change.

5

THE ART OF ADAPTATION: EMBRACING CHANGE

Our bodies, like the seasons, undergo their own transformations as we journey through life. Aging with grace requires us to understand and accept these physical changes. It is a natural part of life that reflects the lives we've lived and the experiences we've valued. However, embracing this new phase can be as challenging as it is inevitable.

Everyone experiences physical change in different ways. Some may notice a difference in strength and stamina, while others may observe changes in skin texture or hair color. Our vision and hearing might not be as sharp as they once were, and we may find ourselves adjusting the font size on our devices or asking others to speak up a bit more often.

Recognizing and accepting these changes does not mean resignation. It means acknowledging the natural course of life and adapting our lifestyles to maintain our health and well-being. It's about finding new ways to stay active that accommodate our changing bodies. Perhaps the long runs of our youth transition into brisk walks or gentle yoga sessions. It's about nourishing our bodies with the right foods, rich in nutrients, that support our vitality at every age.

Understanding our physical changes involves a compassionate dialogue with ourselves. It's about looking in the mirror and seeing beyond the lines and gray hairs to the wisdom and stories they represent. It's about celebrating the body that has allowed us to experience the world in its full splendor and continues to do so, albeit at a different pace.

In this acceptance, there is a quiet strength. It's the strength to ask for help when simple tasks become challenging and the courage to adapt our environments to our needs—through assistive devices or home modifications. It's the strength to share our vulnerabilities with loved ones, fostering deeper connections and mutual support.

Adapting to our physical changes, we pave the way for mental adaptability. Staying flexible in our thoughts and attitudes becomes just as important as maintaining flexibility in our joints. The grace with which we accept our physical selves feeds into the resilience of our minds, allowing us to approach each new day with curiosity and openness.

In the next steps of our journey, we will explore the mental landscape of aging, understanding that our thoughts and attitudes can either be our greatest allies or our most challenging obstacles. As we adapt physically, let us also prepare to cultivate mental adaptability, embracing the full spectrum of changes that come with time.

Mental Adaptability: Staying Flexible

Let's now explore the landscape of the mind, where adaptability and flexibility become our allies in the art of aging with grace.

Mental adaptability is embracing change with an open heart and an agile mind. It is about cultivating a mindset that welcomes transformation as a natural part of life. As we age, our cognitive processes may shift, and our perspectives may evolve, but this does not signify an end to growth. Instead, it presents an opportunity for new learning and different ways of engaging with the world.

We must challenge ourselves to remain curious and open to new ideas to stay mentally flexible. It can be as simple as taking up a new hobby, learning a new language, or engaging in regular intellectual discussions with friends or family. These activities stimulate the brain, fostering neural plasticity, the brain's remarkable ability to reorganize itself by forming new neural connections throughout life.

Another aspect of mental adaptability is the practice of mindfulness. Mindfulness encourages us to live in the present moment and to observe our thoughts and feelings without judgment. This practice can help us navigate the emotional landscape of aging, allowing us to acknowledge and accept our feelings of loss, joy, or anything in between. By being present, we can appreciate the richness of each moment, even as we acknowledge the changes that come with time.

Resilience, too, plays a pivotal role in mental adaptability. Life can sometimes present challenges that test our emotional and psychological limits. As we explored in earlier chapters, building resilience involves developing coping strategies that help us bounce back from adversity. It is about finding strength in vulnerability and learning that it is okay to ask for help when needed. Support networks, whether they consist of family, friends, or community resources, can provide the encouragement and assistance necessary to navigate life's more turbulent waters.

Mental flexibility requires accepting change and embracing it with wisdom and courage. It is about understanding that each new chapter of life brings the potential for growth, discovery, and a deeper appreciation for the mosaic of experiences that define our unique journey through the years.

We must also consider the spaces we inhabit. Our environment plays a significant role in our well-being. As such, the next focus of our journey will be on how we can adjust our living spaces to cater to our changing needs and desires. By harmonizing our external surroundings with our internal states, we create a sanctuary that accommodates our physical requirements and nourishes our mental and emotional health.

Home and Environment: Adjusting Your Living Space

Our homes are often more than just physical spaces; they are repositories of memories, comfort, and personal expression. However, as we age, we may need to reconsider the suitability of our living spaces. The art of adaptation is not only about adjusting our mindset but also about ensuring our environments continue to support our evolving needs.

Changing your living space is a way to take care of yourself. It means recognizing the changes in our lives and taking steps to meet those new needs. This can be both liberating and daunting, but it's an important step towards aging gracefully and keeping your independence.

Firstly, consider the layout of your home. Does it support your current lifestyle and mobility? You might find that rearranging furniture to create wider walkways can make navigation easier. Creating a single-level living space can be ideal, but if that's not possible, ensuring that essential facilities, like a bathroom and a space to sleep, are accessible without having to navigate stairs can be a practical compromise.

Floors should be a focus as well. Slip-resistant flooring can safeguard against falls, a leading cause of injury for older adults. Removing or securing rugs with non-slip pads and choosing carpets with a low pile can also help prevent trips and slips.

It's also worth considering the accessibility of everyday items. Placing frequently used objects within easy reach can minimize strain and the need for unnecessary stretching or bending.

Lighting also plays a crucial role in a comfortable living environment. As our eyes age, we may need more light to see clearly. Assess the lighting in your home, and consider adding brighter bulbs and additional light sources where necessary, especially in areas like stairways and hallways where good visibility is crucial.

In the bathroom, where water and hard surfaces pose a significant risk, installing grab bars by the toilet and shower can provide stability and support. A shower seat and a hand-held showerhead can add comfort and reduce the need to stand for prolonged periods. For some, transitioning to a walk-in bathtub or a zero-threshold shower can be a game-changer, blending accessibility with elegance.

In the kitchen, adjusting the height of counters and sinks to accommodate seated use and ensuring that appliances are easily accessible can make daily tasks easier. Lever-style faucet handles and D-shaped cabinet pulls can simplify cooking and cleaning for those with limited hand strength or dexterity.

Staircases, too, can be made safer with sturdy handrails on both sides and a stairlift if navigating the stairs becomes a challenge. Simple organizational changes, like keeping frequently used items within easy reach, can make a significant difference in daily living.

Our emotional connection to specific items or furniture arrangements may make change difficult. However, the goal is to create a space that is not only safe and functional but also one that continues to feel like home. This might mean finding new ways to display cherished mementos or repurposing rooms to suit your hobbies and activities better.

In making these adjustments, involving family, friends, or a professional specializing in age-friendly home design is beneficial. They can offer insights and help execute changes that align with your vision for a comfortable, accessible living space.

Remember, modifying your home is not about erasing the past or admitting your limitations; it's about shaping your environment to fit the vibrant life you continue to lead. It's proof of your adaptability and a pledge to your health as you face the future with hope and elegance.

As we move forward, it's equally important to stay connected with the evolving world around us. The next step in our adaptation journey involves technology, which, when embraced, can enhance our quality of life and keep us engaged with the world.

Technology: Keeping Up with the Times

The fast speed of tech changes can often seem overwhelming. However, getting comfortable with technology can lead to more freedom and a better connection with the world. Learning to use technology is an art of adjusting that can be achieved with patience and willingness to learn.

The digital age has brought about changes that can be both empowering and overwhelming. The key is to approach technology as a tool, not a barrier. It is a means to stay informed, connected, and engaged with our loved ones and the community.

Learning to use new devices and platforms can feel like learning a new language. Still, it's a language that enables us to share stories, view pictures of our grandchildren, and even manage our health. Video calls can shrink the miles between us and our families, and smart devices can remind us to take medication or track our steps for a healthier lifestyle.

Keeping up with technology does not mean chasing every new gadget or trend. Instead, it's about identifying the technologies that add value to our lives. Whether it's a smartphone that helps us stay in touch, a tablet for reading and games, or a home assistant that makes daily tasks easier, each device should serve a purpose that resonates with your needs and interests.

For those who might feel hesitant, remember that learning is a process. Numerous resources, from community classes to online tutorials, cater to all levels of expertise. Family members and friends can also help you on this journey, offering support and companionship as you explore the digital landscape together.

Technology can also offer a sense of safety and security. With medical alert systems and GPS tracking, we can have the peace of mind that help is available at the push of a button. Smart home technologies can automate lighting, heating, and security, ensuring our environment adapts to our needs without requiring constant attention.

As we integrate technology into our lives, remember to maintain a balance. It should never replace the warmth of human contact or the joy of real-world experiences. Instead, let technology enhance how we live, bringing convenience and connection, but always in harmony with the simple pleasures we've always cherished.

In this art of adaptation, we find that when approached with curiosity and a willingness to learn, technology can be a faithful companion on the journey of aging with grace. It allows us to keep up with the times while holding onto the essence of what makes each moment precious.

The Power of Routine: Finding Comfort in Consistency

With age comes a profound beauty in the regularity of daily routines. These routines stitch together the pattern of our everyday life, giving us a comforting structure as we face the natural changes of aging. They're like familiar tunes that provide a rhythm to our changing lives, allowing our days to move smoothly and gracefully.

Over time, routines often become cherished rituals that allow us to maintain a sense of self and purpose. In the quiet moments of morning tea or the evening stroll, their rhythm resonates with our past, present, and future heartbeats.

The strength of routine is that it both anchors and frees us. It gives us a stable structure in life's sea of uncertainties. This isn't about being inflexible; it's about having a framework that brings peace and steadiness. It's like a comforting hand on our shoulder, reminding us that some things stay the same, even as everything else changes.

At the same time, routines liberate us. They free up mental space by reducing the decisions we need to make, allowing us to conserve our energy for the things that truly matter. This is especially poignant in our later years, when we may wish to focus on nurturing relationships, exploring new hobbies, or simply savoring the quiet beauty of the world around us.

However, routines are not set in stone; they are adaptable. As our needs and circumstances change, so too can our routines. This adaptability is key to aging with grace. It is about finding the balance between the comfort of the familiar and the thrill of the new.

In embracing the power of routine, we also embrace the power of self-care. Each step in our daily routine can be an act of kindness towards ourselves. From the nourishing meals we prepare to the restorative sleep we prioritize, each element of our routine is a building block in the temple of our well-being.

Don't underestimate the profound simplicity of a daily routine. They protect our days and care for our well-being quietly. In the art of aging, we should cherish them, as they are the faithful companions that walk alongside us through life's ever-changing seasons.

Chapter Summary

- Aging gracefully involves understanding and accepting the physical changes that come with time, such as decreased strength and changes in vision and hearing.
- Adapting to these changes means finding new ways to stay active, eating nutritious foods, and having a compassionate dialogue with oneself.
- Mental adaptability is crucial as we age, involving staying curious, learning new things, practicing mindfulness, and building resilience.
- Adjusting living spaces to accommodate aging is a form of self-care that may involve changes to your home layout, lighting, and assistive devices.

- Embracing technology can enhance independence and connection with others, and it's important to find a balance and choose technologies that add value.
- Routines provide a comforting sense of order and familiarity, helping to conserve energy for what matters most. They can be adapted to changing needs and circumstances, allowing for both stability and the incorporation of new experiences.
- Daily routines are acts of self-care and can be essential for maintaining well-being as we age.

6

SELF-CARE AND INDEPENDENCE

As we age, the value of daily self-care becomes clearer. It's essential for maintaining our physical health, emotional wellness, and independence. Self-care isn't a luxury; it's a vital set of practices that help us age gracefully and with dignity.

At the heart of daily self-care is personal hygiene. This covers a range of activities from bathing to oral care, each playing a vital role in fostering a sense of self-respect and confidence. Regular bathing refreshes the body, stimulates circulation, and provides a time for self-reflection and relaxation. On the other hand, oral care is crucial for preventing discomfort and maintaining the ability to enjoy a variety of foods.

Nutrition is another form of self-care. As we age, our bodies' needs change, and so must our diets. As we learned in earlier chapters, prioritizing nutrient-dense foods, staying hydrated, and being mindful of portion sizes help maintain energy levels and support bodily functions. It's also about the dining experience, which should be pleasurable and, when possible, a social activity that connects us with others.

Physical activity, tailored to individual ability and preference, is another non-negotiable aspect of self-care. Whether it's a gentle walk, a series of stretches, or a yoga class, regular movement is essential for preserving flexibility, strength, and balance. It also has profound effects on mental health, helping to alleviate stress and promote a positive mood.

Rest is equally important. Quality sleep is restorative, helping to repair the body and consolidate memories. Establishing a regular sleep routine, creating a comfortable sleeping environment, and promptly addressing any sleep disturbances with a healthcare provider are all critical steps in ensuring that rest is a rejuvenating part of daily life.

Mental and emotional care is as important as physical care. Engaging in activities that stimulate the mind, such as reading, puzzles, or learning new skills, helps to keep the brain active and resilient. Equally important is nurturing emotional health by maintaining social connections, seeking laughter and joy, and finding ways to express feelings and thoughts through conversation, writing, or other creative outlets.

Self-care also includes managing health care. This means being proactive about medical appointments, understanding and adhering to prescribed treatments, and maintaining open communication with healthcare providers. It involves being informed and making decisions that align with your values and quality of life.

In embracing these non-negotiables of daily self-care, we honor our present selves and lay the framework for continued independence and quality of life as we age. These daily acts of self-care can help us navigate the changes of aging with more resilience and grace.

Mobility and Accessibility: Tools for Independence

Our needs for getting around and accessing things may evolve over time. This natural change requires us to adapt, not to give up our independence. With the right aids and environmental changes, we can keep moving through our daily lives confidently and independently.

Mobility aids can be a key to maintaining freedom. A well-chosen walking stick can be a trusted companion on strolls, providing stability and reducing the load on weary joints. For those who find greater comfort in additional support, walkers or rollators offer a sturdy frame to lean on, often equipped with seats and baskets that invite rest and carry personal items during outings.

For longer distances or when energy reserves are low, wheelchairs or mobility scooters can be helpful modes of transport. These tools empower us to participate in family gatherings, community events, and outdoor adventures without worrying about tiredness. If you are considering investing in one of these, select a model that aligns with your lifestyle, ensuring it is comfortable and capable of navigating the spaces you frequently wander.

Adapting our homes is equally crucial in fostering independence. Ramps can replace steps, creating smooth transitions from outdoors to indoors. Doorways may be widened to accommodate mobility aids, and thresholds can be minimized to prevent tripping hazards. Smart home devices enable us to control lighting and temperature and even lock doors with the sound of our voice or the touch of a button. These advancements bring peace of mind and reduce the physical strain of household tasks.

Adopting these tools does not diminish our capabilities but rather enhances them. They are not markers of limitations but symbols of our resourcefulness and determination to live on our terms. By embracing mobility and accessibility tools, we make a conscious choice to age with grace, ensuring that our environment adapts to us as much as we adapt.

Personal Safety: Feeling Secure in Your Environment

During this time, our homes become increasingly important as places of comfort and security. The walls that have seen years of emotions and experiences now protect our daily tranquility and safety. Personal safety, often forgotten, is a key part of self-care and keeping our independence as we grow older.

Feeling secure in your environment is not just about locks on the doors or the brightness of outdoor lights; it's about creating a living space that respects your needs and anticipates potential risks. It's about fostering a sense of well-being from knowing you are protected and prepared for the unexpected.

Technology can be a helpful ally in personal safety. Emergency response systems can be worn as pendants or watches, providing a direct line to assistance should you need it. These devices are designed to be unobtrusive and empowering, giving you and your loved ones peace of mind.

But personal safety extends beyond the physical. It's also about feeling secure knowing you have a support network. This network could include family, friends, neighbors, or community services aware of your routines and ready to offer help if your pattern changes unexpectedly. Regular check-ins can be arranged, not as a sign of frailty, but as a proactive approach to staying connected and secure.

In addition to a support network, consider the role of local authorities and community resources. Familiarize yourself with their services, such as neighborhood watch programs or senior safety initiatives. These resources can provide valuable information and assistance, reinforcing the safety net around you.

Lastly, personal safety is deeply intertwined with emotional well-being. A home that feels secure is a space where stress is minimized and relaxation is invited. It's a place where you can move freely, without fear, and sleep soundly, knowing that you have taken steps to ensure your safety and independence.

By integrating these strategies into your daily life, you create not just a house but a home that supports and protects you through the years.

Managing Medications: A Guide to Responsible Use

In our golden years, taking care of ourselves often involves managing different medications, each with its role and significance. Using these medications responsibly is crucial for keeping our health and independence. It's a careful balance that needs focus, good management, and, sometimes, a bit of wisdom.

Understanding the medications you are prescribed is fundamental. Each medication has a role to play in your well-being, and being informed about their effects, side effects, why you're taking them and how they interact with each other is vital. Do not hesitate to ask your healthcare provider questions about your medications. They can give you the knowledge to take your medications safely and effectively.

Organization is your friend when it comes to managing medications. A pill organizer can be a simple yet effective tool, helping track what needs to be taken and when. Some organizers come with compartments for different times of the day, which can be particularly helpful if your medication regimen is complex. Maintaining a medication list that includes dosages, times, and special instructions can be invaluable, especially if you need to visit a healthcare provider unfamiliar with your medical history.

Adherence to your medication schedule is as important as the medications themselves. Missing doses or taking them at the wrong time can diminish their effectiveness and potentially put your health at risk. If you find remembering to take your medications challenging, consider setting alarms on a clock, watch, or smartphone. There are also apps designed to help manage medication schedules, providing reminders and tracking your adherence over time.

Monitoring for side effects is another aspect of responsible medication management. While medications are intended to help you, they can sometimes cause adverse reactions. Be vigilant about any changes in how you feel after starting a new medication or changing a dose. If you notice anything unusual, report it to your healthcare provider promptly. They can determine if what you are experiencing is expected or adjustments must be made.

Lastly, regular reviews of your medications with your healthcare provider are essential. As your body changes with age, so can how it responds to medications. A once-suitable medication may become less so over time, or new options may be available that could work better for you. These reviews are also an opportunity to check that all of your medications are still necessary and to eliminate any that are not, reducing the risk of polypharmacy.

As you continue to curate the narrative of your life, remember that asking for help when needed is not a sign of weakness but rather a wise acknowledgment of the complexity of self-care.

Asking for Help: Balancing Independence and Support

Taking care of ourselves often means balancing staying independent and knowing when to ask for help. This balance changes as our abilities and situations change. As we grow older, it's essential to understand that seeking help isn't a weakness but a sign of strength and wisdom.

Independence is a cherished value that provides a sense of control, dignity, and purpose. It's understandable to cling to it tightly, as it forms a core part of our identity. However, life's natural progression may lead to moments when self-sufficiency becomes challenging. This is where interdependence may be required—a concept that allows for giving and receiving support to benefit all involved.

To ask for help is to engage in an act of self-care. It requires courage to admit that we cannot do everything alone, and it opens up opportunities for growth and connection. When we allow others to assist us, we not only ease our burdens but also enrich the lives of those who step in to lend a hand.

It's essential to recognize the signs that indicate it might be time to seek assistance. Perhaps managing the household has become more taxing, or personal care routines are not as effortless as they once were. Maybe the complexities of managing medications, as discussed earlier, have highlighted the need for a more structured support system. Whatever the indicators, it's important to assess them honestly and take proactive steps.

One of the most practical approaches to asking for help is understanding your needs clearly. Identifying specific tasks requiring assistance can make the process less overwhelming and more manageable. Communicating openly with loved ones about these needs is beneficial, as they may not always be apparent to others.

When reaching out for help, consider the various resources available. Family and friends are often the first line of support, but there are also community services, professional caregivers, and support groups that can provide the necessary assistance. Explore these options and find what works best for your situation.

In maintaining independence, setting boundaries and expressing preferences is equally important. Accepting help does not mean relinquishing control over your life. It's about making informed choices and directing the type of assistance you want to receive. Doing so allows you to continue leading a life that aligns with your values and desires.

Asking for help is proof of the resilience and adaptability that comes with aging. It's about recognizing the changes in our abilities and adjusting our approach to self-care accordingly. By balancing independence with the proper support, we can continue to live fulfilling lives, moving through our golden years with confidence and respect.

Chapter Summary

- Self-care is an essential part of aging with grace, encompassing personal hygiene, nutrition, physical activity, rest, mental and emotional care, and healthcare management.
- Personal hygiene, including bathing and oral care, boosts confidence and health. At the same time, nutrition may need to be adjusted with age to maintain energy and health.

- Regular physical activity is crucial for maintaining flexibility, strength, balance, and mental health, and quality sleep is restorative for the body and mind.
- Mental and emotional well-being involves stimulating the brain and maintaining social connections while managing healthcare, including proactive medical appointments and treatments.
- Mobility aids and home adaptations, such as ramps and grab bars, can enhance independence, and smart home devices can ease household tasks.
- Personal safety in the home is vital, involving clear pathways, adequate lighting, emergency response systems, and a support network.
- Responsible medication management requires understanding, organization, adherence, monitoring for side effects, and regular reviews with healthcare providers.
- Asking for help is a strength, not a weakness. It involves acknowledging when support is needed, understanding your needs, and finding the right balance of resources and independence.

7

LEISURE AND EXPLORING NEW HORIZONS IN RETIREMENT

As we enter retirement, life offers a range of opportunities, encouraging us to fill our days with the excitement of exploration and learning. Travel at this time isn't just about seeing new places; it's a deep dive into the world's wide variety of cultures, environments, and histories.

Traveling in retirement celebrates the freedom earned after years of hard work, offering a break from the usual and a chance to experience new things. It is an opportunity to step out of the familiar, challenge the mind, and enrich the soul. For many, it's the fulfillment of a long-held dream, an opportunity to see the places they've always wanted to visit that have quietly called to them.

Travel is also a unique chance to reconnect with yourself and your loved ones. It can be a solitary pilgrimage to places with personal significance or a group adventure with family and friends, creating memories that will be cherished for years. It is a time to forge new friendships with people from all walks of life, share stories and laughter, and learn from the collective wisdom of diverse cultures.

The beauty of travel at this stage is the luxury of time. Without the constraints of limited vacation days, you can immerse yourself fully in the experience, whether lingering in a museum to absorb every detail, taking the long route to savor the landscape, or sitting at a café and watching the world go by. This is the time to take things slowly, be present in the moment, and appreciate the small details that a rushed journey might overlook.

Travel can be tailored to the comfort and pace that suits your lifestyle and needs. Many options are available, from leisurely river cruises to guided tours that take care of all the details, allowing travelers to enjoy their adventures without stress or strain.

Travel can also be an enriching conduit for learning and growth. It challenges you to step out of your comfort zone, navigate new languages, taste unfamiliar cuisines, and understand different ways of life. It is an active engagement with the world that keeps the mind sharp and the spirit young.

Exploring hobbies in retirement adds another layer of life satisfaction. While travel broadens our external horizons, hobbies encourage us to look inside ourselves, discovering new aspects of who we are and new paths to happiness and creativity.

Hobbies: The Joy of Personal Passions

In our golden years, we find ourselves with limitless time and a desire for fulfillment. Engaging in hobbies that bring us joy and fuel our passions is an essential part of our overall happiness and health.

Hobbies offer a unique blend of pleasure and purpose, a combination that is especially meaningful during retirement. They allow us to express ourselves, learn and grow, and connect with others on a level that transcends the mundane. Whether it's the delicate art of painting, the rhythmic pleasure of knitting, the challenge of chess, or the physical satisfaction of gardening, hobbies provide a canvas for our creativity and a playground for our intellect.

The beauty of personal passions comes from their variety and the unique significance they have for each person. For some, collecting antiques or stamps offers a connection to history and a sense of continuity. For others, photography captures the fleeting beauty of the world around us, freezing moments in time to be cherished forever.

Engaging in hobbies also has a profound impact on our health. Studies have shown that staying mentally and physically active can lead to a longer and more satisfying life. The concentration required to master a new skill can improve cognitive function, while the social interaction often accompanying hobby groups can ward off loneliness and depression.

Hobbies can also be a form of legacy, a way to share our knowledge and passions with younger generations. The recipes perfected over a lifetime, woodwork crafted with skilled hands, or quilt that weaves together the fabric of family history are gifts that carry a part of ourselves into the future.

Hobbies enrich our lives in numerous ways. Commitment to a hobby can lead to expertise, provide personal fulfillment, and earn the respect and admiration of others. Retirement's flexibility lets us discover new interests or reawaken past passions, reigniting the excitement we felt in our younger days.

Hobbies add color, texture, and pattern to our lives. They remind us that, at any age, happiness can be found in the pursuit of personal passions.

Volunteering: Giving Back with Time and Talent

After exploring the rich satisfaction that hobbies can provide, it's worth considering another avenue of fulfillment that enriches the self and the broader community: volunteering.

Volunteering is a powerful way to give back, a gesture of gratitude, and an act that shows that every individual can make a difference. It's about sharing the most valuable assets one possesses – time and talent – to create positive change. As we age, volunteering offers a unique opportunity to apply a lifetime of skills and knowledge in new, meaningful ways.

The beauty of volunteering lies in its diversity. Opportunities arise in various sectors, including education, healthcare, environmental conservation, and the arts. You might find fulfillment in mentoring young people, bringing your professional expertise to nonprofit organizations, or providing companionship to those in need.

Volunteering has a symbiotic nature. While the main goal is to contribute to the welfare of others, volunteers often find that they receive as much as they give. The social interaction and sense of purpose you can get from volunteering can combat loneliness and depression, common concerns in later life. It can also provide a sense of structure and routine that some people miss after leaving the workforce.

In addition to the emotional and psychological benefits, there's evidence to suggest that volunteering can positively affect physical health. Engaging with others and staying active in a volunteer role can help maintain mental acuity, physical stamina, and overall well-being.

Giving back through volunteering is both a service to the community and a gift to yourself. It's a way to remain connected, continue growing, and acknowledge that no matter your age, there are always new ways to contribute and new joys to discover.

Gardening: The Therapeutic Touch of Nature

As the sun rises, casting a warm glow over soft petals and dewy leaves, a sense of peace and anticipation fills the air. Gardening is a celebration of life, growth, and continual renewal. It's a hobby that combines the beauty of nature with the nurturing touch of our hands, creating a sanctuary where time slows down and the soul is nourished.

For many, gardening is a therapeutic ritual. The feel of soil between your fingers, the careful tending to a budding plant, and watching it flourish can be deeply rewarding. Gardening showcases the virtues of patience and the benefits of careful nurturing. In our later years, it provides a perfect mix of exercise and leisure, a balance crucial if we want to age gracefully.

The garden is a canvas for creativity and expression. Choosing which seeds to plant, designing the layout of a flowerbed, or pairing vegetables and herbs that will grow in harmony all contribute to a sense of purpose and fulfillment. The colors, textures, and fragrances of a garden can be a source of immense pleasure, stimulating the senses in a calming and invigorating way.

Gardening encourages us to connect with the cycles of nature. It teaches us to accept the impermanent nature of life as seasons change and plants go through their life cycles. There's a lesson in witnessing the first sprouts of spring, the abundance of summer, the harvests of autumn, and the quiet dormancy of winter. Each season has its beauty and role in the grand cycle of life.

There are also numerous health benefits of gardening. It's a gentle exercise that can improve endurance, flexibility, and strength. Tasks like digging, planting, weeding, and watering contribute to maintaining physical health without the strain of high-impact activities. Additionally, exposure to sunlight provides essential vitamin D, which is vital for bone health and immune function.

Gardening also offers an opportunity for social interaction and community building. Sharing cuttings, exchanging tips with fellow gardeners, or simply enjoying the company of others in a community garden can lead to meaningful relationships and a sense of belonging. It's a way to stay engaged with others, share in the fruits of harvest, and support each other through nature's challenges.

For those who may not have access to a garden, container gardening is a wonderful alternative. It allows the cultivation of herbs, flowers, and even some vegetables from the comfort of a balcony or windowsill. This adaptability ensures that the therapeutic touch of nature is within reach for everyone, regardless of where they live.

In the tranquility of the garden, there is a space for reflection and meditation. It's a place where the world's worries can be set aside, and the focus can shift to the simple, grounding tasks at hand. Gardening is a reminder that growth and change are constants. As we cultivate our gardens, we also cultivate our well-being, finding joy in the rhythm of nature and the simple act of nurturing life.

Games and Recreation: Fun as a Fountain of Youth

In retirement, seeking leisure and fun is an essential part of a lively and satisfying life. Games and recreation aren't just for children; they're like a source of youthfulness, helping to keep our minds and bodies agile and spirited.

Games offer a unique blend of mental stimulation and social interaction that can be particularly beneficial as we age. Board games, card games, and even digital games can sharpen cognitive skills, enhance memory, and foster problem-solving abilities. Engaging in these playful challenges can be a great way to keep the brain active and engaged and help ward off the mental fog that sometimes accompanies aging.

Recreational activities like bowling, dancing, or even participating in a local theater production can provide physical exercise and a sense of community and belonging. These activities encourage us to step out of our comfort zones, learn new skills, and connect with others, all of which are essential for aging gracefully.

Laughter and joy that inherently come with games and recreation are powerful antidotes to stress and loneliness. They remind us that life can be filled with fun and playfulness at any age. In these times of fun and friendship, we often discover the strongest bonds with our friends, family, and even within ourselves.

If you integrate games and recreational activities into your daily routine, you'll discover that they are more than simply a way to pass the time. They celebrate life's continued potential for growth, learning, and happiness. They are a way to embrace fun as a fundamental part of our lives. Through these different experiences, we continue to evolve, proving that we are all young at heart, no matter our age.

Chapter Summary

- Retirement offers the opportunity to travel, providing a meaningful engagement with diverse cultures and the freedom to explore long-held dreams. It allows us to reconnect with ourselves and loved ones, creating cherished memories and new friendships.
- Hobbies are a source of joy and self-expression, offering a chance to pursue personal passions and stay

mentally and physically active. Engaging in hobbies can improve health, provide a sense of purpose, and allow us to leave a legacy through shared knowledge and skills.

- Volunteering during retirement enables us to give back to the community, utilizing our time and talents in meaningful ways. It offers emotional, psychological, and physical health benefits, fostering social connections and a sense of purpose.
- Gardening can provide therapeutic benefits, physical activity, and a connection to nature, contributing to overall well-being and community engagement.
- Games and recreational activities in later years promote mental agility, social interaction, and physical activity, enhancing quality of life and fostering a youthful spirit.

8

HEALTH CHALLENGES AND MEDICAL CARE

As we age, figuring out the healthcare system is like navigating a new terrain with an intricate map. The prospect can be daunting at first, but with the right knowledge and support, it can also be a journey to maintaining and enhancing our quality of life.

Understanding the healthcare system is crucial because it is the gateway to receiving the medical care and support we need. This system is more than just a collection of doctors and hospitals; it's a complex network of insurance plans, pharmacies, specialists, and home health services, all of which are there to help us stay on top of our health as we age.

One of the first steps in navigating this system with ease is to establish a strong relationship with a primary care physician. This doctor will become your main point of contact, helping to coordinate care and make informed decisions about your health. They are the ones who know your medical history, understand your concerns, and can help you out when specialists or additional services are needed.

We often find ourselves managing multiple prescriptions with age. It can be helpful to have a pharmacist you trust to discuss your medications, their possible side effects, and how they interact. A good pharmacist can be a valuable resource, offering advice on medication management and ensuring that your treatment plan is safe and effective.

Insurance is another aspect of the healthcare system that can be particularly complex. Understanding your coverage, what it entails, and how to maximize your benefits is a skill that will serve you well. Don't hesitate to ask questions or seek assistance from insurance representatives or patient advocacy groups to clarify your entitlements and responsibilities.

Technology has also become a significant part of healthcare management. From online patient portals that allow you to access your medical records to telehealth services that enable you to consult with doctors virtually, don't be afraid to embrace these tools. They can simplify managing appointments, refilling prescriptions, and keeping track of your health.

Support groups and community services can offer invaluable assistance. These groups provide practical advice and assistance as well as emotional support from others who understand the challenges of aging. Whether it's help with transportation to medical appointments or navigating health-related paperwork, these organizations can be a lifeline.

Lastly, remember that you are not alone on this journey. Family, friends, and caregivers can be integral in helping you manage your healthcare needs. They can accompany you to appointments, help you manage medication, or be there to listen when you're feeling overwhelmed.

Navigating the healthcare system as we age can be challenging but can be met with grace and determination. By building a network of trusted professionals, staying informed, and getting support when needed, we can take control of our health and continue to live life to the fullest.

Chronic Conditions: Managing Long-Term Health Issues

Chronic health conditions can often feel like an unwelcome companion on our path through life. These long-term health issues, which may include arthritis, hypertension, diabetes, heart disease, and osteoporosis, among others, are conditions that we need to understand and handle with patience and kindness.

Managing chronic conditions involves balancing medical advice with personal lifestyle choices. It begins with a comprehensive understanding of each condition, its potential complications, and available treatments. Knowledge is empowering; when armed with the right information, you can make informed decisions about your health care.

Regular check-ups and open communication with doctors can help monitor the progress of these conditions and adjust treatments if needed. It is important to ask questions, express your concerns, and discuss any side effects of medications or therapies. Remember, you are the most important member of your healthcare team, and your insights into your body's responses are invaluable.

Lifestyle modifications also play a significant role in managing chronic conditions. A balanced diet, regular physical activity, and adequate rest are foundational to maintaining health and vitality. Nutritional needs can change with age, so it may be beneficial to consult with a dietitian to ensure that your diet supports your health conditions. Similarly, appropriate exercise can help manage symptoms and improve overall well-being. Even gentle activities like walking, swimming, or tai chi can make a significant difference.

Emotional support is just as important as physical care. Chronic conditions can sometimes lead to feelings of frustration, isolation, or sadness. Seek support from friends, family, or support groups where experiences and coping strategies can be shared. Remember, you are not alone on this journey, and sharing your story can provide comfort and offer others insights.

Aging with grace while managing chronic conditions is about embracing each day with optimism and resilience. It's about making informed choices, seeking joy in the everyday, and recognizing the beauty in the wisdom that comes with experience.

Mental Health Concerns: Addressing Depression and Anxiety

We've already explored the importance of looking after our bodies and minds. Our lives are full of experiences, but sometimes, as we age, we might start to struggle with our mental health, facing challenges like depression and anxiety. These aren't just small worries that come and go; they're bigger issues that can impact how happy and comfortable we feel every day. We should take these concerns seriously and treat them with as much care and kindness as a physical illness.

Depression in the later stages of life is often misinterpreted as a natural part of aging, but this is not always true. Depression is not an inevitable consequence of growing older but a medical condition that can and should be treated. The symptoms may be subtle or mistakenly attributed to other health issues or life changes, such as losing loved ones, retirement, or physical decline. However, it can significantly impact one's sense of joy, energy, and purpose, which can be immense.

Similarly, anxiety can be a silent but heavy burden, making us worry about health, financial security, and the well-being of family members. It can manifest as a constant sense of nervousness, trouble sleeping, or feeling overwhelmed by small, everyday tasks.

The first step in addressing these mental health concerns is recognition. We need to listen to ourselves with the same empathy we offer others. Acknowledging feelings of sadness, worry, or fear is an act of courage, not a sign of weakness. Have open conversations with healthcare providers, who can offer screenings and referrals to mental health professionals if needed.

Treatment for depression and anxiety can take many forms, and each person may face it differently. Medication can be an effective tool, but it is often most beneficial when combined with other therapies. Counseling or psychotherapy provides a space to explore feelings and develop coping strategies. Cognitive-behavioral therapy, in particular, has shown promise in helping older adults reframe negative thought patterns that contribute to depression and anxiety.

Beyond clinical interventions, there are everyday actions that can boost your mental health. Maintaining social connections, engaging in physical activity if your health permits, and cultivating hobbies and interests can all play a role in lifting spirits and reducing anxiety. Mindfulness practices, such as meditation or deep-breathing exercises, can also be powerful allies in the quest for mental tranquility.

It's also important to consider the environment in which one ages. A supportive community, whether family, friends, or a dedicated senior living arrangement, can provide the social stimulation and sense of belonging that are vital to mental health. Access to resources such as senior centers, support groups, and educational workshops can empower older adults to take charge of their mental well-being.

Mental health is not a destination but a continuous path we walk, with its own set of challenges and triumphs. By addressing conditions like depression and anxiety with the same care we give to physical illnesses, we honor the full spectrum of our health and embrace the possibility of a life lived with happiness and resilience.

HANNA BENTSEN

Rehabilitation and Recovery: Bouncing Back from Illness

Our strength and spirit are often tested by the health challenges that come with age. No one wants illness, but it doesn't have to be a permanent resident in our lives. The road to recovery, though sometimes tough and full of twists and turns, is paved with the promise of rehabilitation and the chance of returning to a life of purpose and happiness.

Rehabilitation, often associated with strength and renewal, is vital to the healing process. It is the bridge that carries us from sickness to health. For older people, it's not only about physical recovery. It's about reclaiming independence, maintaining self-respect, and making their lives more enjoyable.

The process of rehabilitation and recovery is different for everyone. It usually starts with a comprehensive assessment by healthcare professionals who understand the situation. This team could include physicians, nurses, physical therapists, occupational therapists, speech therapists, and social workers, all working together to tailor a recovery plan that respects the individual's goals and limitations.

Physical therapy is crucial in helping us regain strength, balance, and mobility in our later years. It provides the adage that movement is medicine. Through guided exercises and encouragement, physical therapists help individuals rebuild the physical abilities that may have been eroded by illness. On the other hand, occupational therapy focuses on the practical aspects of daily living, ensuring that individuals can navigate their environments safely and perform the tasks that bring meaning to their lives.

Speech therapy is also an essential part of the recovery process for those facing neurological events or other communication conditions. The ability to express oneself and engage in conversation is a cornerstone of human connection, and speech therapists work diligently to restore this critical aspect of interaction.

The emotional and psychological dimensions of recovery are equally important. Returning to good health can be overloaded with frustration, fear, and uncertainty. Here, the compassionate support of mental health professionals and loved ones becomes invaluable, helping support the spirit as the body heals.

Rehabilitation thrives on the support system surrounding the individual—family, friends, and caregivers offering their presence as a source of comfort and motivation. Their involvement is often the catalyst that propels recovery forward, transforming the rehabilitation experience into a shared journey.

Technology has brought new dimensions to rehabilitation, with innovative tools and devices enhancing the therapeutic experience. From telemedicine consultations to advanced equipment that aids in physical therapy, technology has become a powerful tool in the journey to recovery.

As individuals progress through rehabilitation, it is essential to celebrate each milestone, no matter how small. These victories are the stepping stones that lead to a fuller, more active life. They are reminders that every effort invested in recovery shows the enduring strength of the human spirit.

The determination to recover and the support of a caring community ultimately guide us back to the rhythm of life. The path of rehabilitation and recovery is one of transformation, where each step taken is closer to regaining the independence and well-being that enables us to live life to the fullest.

End-of-Life Care: Understanding Your Options

At some point in our lives, we are confronted with the reality that life is a cycle with a beginning and an end. Accepting this cycle with grace means acknowledging and preparing for the final stage of life. End-of-life care is a sensitive and important topic that deserves our attention and understanding. It includes the medical and emotional support provided during the period leading up to death. The goal is to make sure they are comfortable, their choices are respected, and their life is as good as it can be during this time.

Understanding your options for end-of-life care is an act of compassion for your loved ones. It involves making decisions that may be difficult but are essential in ensuring that your values and desires are honored. One of the primary options to consider is hospice care, which is designed to offer a supportive environment for individuals in the final phases of a terminal illness. Hospice care prioritizes pain management and emotional support, providing services at home, a hospice center, or a hospital.

Palliative care is another option that focuses on providing relief from the symptoms and stress of a severe illness. The goal is to improve the patients' and families' quality of life. Palliative care can be provided alongside curative treatments and is not limited to those at the end of life.

As we explored earlier, advance directives are legal documents that allow you to outline your preferences for end-of-life care before you cannot communicate them. These include a living will, which specifies the types of medical treatment you wish to receive or avoid, and a power of attorney for health care, which designates a person to make decisions on your behalf if you are unable to.

The conversation about end-of-life care is a very personal one. It involves discussing your wishes with family and healthcare providers, ensuring everyone understands your values and preferences. These discussions can provide peace of mind for you and your loved ones, knowing that your choices will be respected.

It's also essential to consider the emotional and spiritual aspects of end-of-life care. Many find comfort in counseling, spiritual guidance, or simply the presence of family and friends. Creating a peaceful environment, filled with personal touches like favorite music or cherished photographs, can also be a part of this final chapter.

In navigating these choices, seek healthcare professionals experienced in end-of-life care who can provide the guidance and support you need. They can help you understand the implications of different care options and help coordinate the various aspects of end-of-life care.

Chapter Summary

- The healthcare system can seem daunting at times, involving doctors, insurance, pharmacies, and home health services. Establishing a relationship with a primary care physician can help you coordinate your care and make health decisions.
- Trusting pharmacists can help manage medications and understand their interactions and side effects.
- Understanding insurance coverage and benefits is crucial; technology can help manage health records and appointments.
- Family, friends, and caregivers are vital in assisting with healthcare management, while support groups and community services can provide additional practical and emotional support as we age.
- Managing chronic conditions involves understanding the conditions, working with healthcare providers, and making lifestyle changes that suit you.
- Addressing mental health, such as depression and anxiety, is just as important as dealing with physical

illness. Treatments for mental health conditions include medication, therapy, and social support.
- End-of-life care is a sensitive and important topic that deserves attention and understanding. It includes the medical and emotional support provided during the period leading up to death and discussing your wishes with family and healthcare providers to ensure everyone understands your values and preferences.

9

THE DIGITAL AGE: STAYING CONNECTED AND INFORMED

The ways we connect with others and learn new things get more complex and colorful as technology advances. The internet, a vast and ever-expanding digital universe, offers many resources that can enrich our lives in countless ways. The internet is a way to connect to the wider world, a library of endless knowledge, and a space to share our stories and experiences.

From the comfort of your home, you can access a world of

resources to help you stay informed, learn new skills, and even manage your daily life more easily. Online banking, for instance, simplifies the way we handle our finances, allowing us to pay bills and monitor our accounts without the need to queue at the bank. Health portals provide valuable insights into wellness and medical information, empowering us to take charge of our health with informed decisions.

Online courses and tutorials allow us to learn anything, no matter where we are. Whether picking up a new language, exploring the mysteries of the universe, or delving into the arts, the internet is an ever-present mentor ready to guide you through your learning journey. It is a place where the mind can remain sharp and engaged, and the pursuit of knowledge continues to kindle the spirit of lifelong learning.

The internet is also a treasure trove of entertainment and leisure. Streaming services bring the thrill of cinema and television series into our living rooms, offering an escape to other worlds and stories. E-books and audiobooks provide a refuge for book lovers, ensuring that the joy of reading is only a click away.

Navigating this digital realm may seem scary initially, but with patience and a willingness to learn, it becomes a rewarding extension of one's living space. Approach the internet with a sense of adventure and openness, balanced with a healthy awareness of online safety and privacy. By setting strong passwords, understanding the basics of internet security, and being careful about the information we share, we can navigate the digital world safely and with confidence.

As we embrace the internet's vast offerings, we find that it keeps us connected not only to the world but also to our evolving selves. It fulfills the human need for growth and adaptation, proving that no matter our age, we can continue to expand our horizons and enrich our lives with the resources at our fingertips.

Social Media: Keeping in Touch with Loved Ones

Social media, often perceived as the young's playground, can also be a sanctuary for us as we navigate the golden years. It is a bridge across generations, a meeting place where grandparents can witness the milestones of their grandchildren, old friends can reunite with the ease of a click, and wisdom can be shared with the world.

The beauty of social media lies in its ability to adapt to our needs. For those who have watched the world evolve and seen the birth of television and the rise of the internet, social media is not just another technological leap; it is a tool that can be molded to fit the contours of their lives. It allows the sharing of stories, the celebration of anniversaries, and the comfort of seeing a loved one's face, even if they are miles away.

Engaging with these platforms can be as straightforward or as involved as one desires. You can start by creating a profile on a platform that resonates with you, be it the visual stories of Instagram, the community conversations of Facebook, or the rapid-fire updates of Twitter. Approach these spaces with curiosity and an open heart.

Privacy and comfort are paramount, and social media can be tailored to respect these boundaries. Customizing privacy settings ensures you share your life with those you trust, creating a safe space to express yourself. It's also a place to listen, learn from the experiences of others, and engage in the global dialogue that shapes our world.

If you're worried about the complexities of these platforms, fear not. The intuitive design of most social media sites makes them accessible, and there is always help at hand, be it from family, friends, or the platforms' support systems. The initial steps into this digital realm can be taken slowly, and with each venture, confidence grows. It's not about keeping pace with the changing algorithms or the latest trends; it's about finding a rhythm that suits your beat.

As we age, the desire to remain part of the community, to be involved and informed, continues. Social media offers that continuity, ensuring the world does not drift away as the years pass. It is both a window to the world and a mirror reflecting the life you've lived and the life you continue to live.

In this digital age, aging with grace includes embracing the tools that allow us to stay connected and informed. If you wish, carry the essence of who you are into the virtual realm and find joy in the new ways you can remain interwoven in those around you. As we continue our journey through the chapters of life, remember that the heart does not grow old. Its beat can be heard through social media across the vast expanse of the digital world.

Online Security: Protecting Yourself in the Digital World

Embracing the digital world brings a wealth of opportunities to stay connected and informed. However, as we navigate this ever-evolving landscape, we must be vigilant about our online security. While a tool of immense utility, the internet can also be a playground for those with less than honorable intentions. As we age, protecting our digital presence becomes even more critical to safeguard our personal information and ensure that our online experiences remain positive and enriching.

First and foremost, understand the basics of online security. This begins with the creation of strong, unique passwords for each of your accounts. A strong password is like a sturdy lock on the door of your online home; it should be complex, including a mix of letters, numbers, and symbols, and it should be changed regularly. Consider using a reputable password manager to keep track of your passwords, as this can alleviate the burden of memorization while maintaining a high level of security.

Another key aspect of online security is recognizing and avoiding phishing attempts. Phishing is a deceptive practice where scammers send emails or messages that appear to be from legitimate sources, such as your bank or a familiar service provider, to trick you into revealing sensitive information. Always be cautious with emails requesting personal details or urging you to click on unfamiliar links. When in doubt, contact the company directly using a phone number or website address you trust.

Updating your software is another simple yet effective step in protecting yourself online. Updates often include security patches that close vulnerabilities in your software, making it harder for hackers to access your system. Set your devices to update automatically, or make it a habit to check for updates regularly.

Socializing online can be a delightful way to keep in touch with friends and family, but it's important to manage your privacy settings on social media platforms. Customize who can see your posts and personal information. Be selective about what you share, and remember that the internet has a long memory; once something is posted, it can be difficult to erase.

Lastly, consider using two-factor authentication wherever possible. This adds an extra layer of security by requiring a second form of verification, such as a code sent to your phone, in addition to your password. This means that even if someone were to discover your password, they would still need this second code to access your account.

Taking these precautions can reduce the risk of falling victim to online threats. Staying informed about the latest security measures is as important as staying connected.

Smart Devices: Simplifying Daily Tasks

Embracing technology can enhance daily living rather than complicate it. Smart devices, with their intuitive interfaces and customizable features, offer many ways to simplify the tasks that once demanded more of our time and physical effort.

Imagine a morning that begins not with the arduous task of wrestling with appliance manuals or the physical strain of reaching high shelves but with a simple voice command that brews your coffee, adjusts the thermostat, or even reminds you to take your medication. This is the world smart devices have ushered in, where aging does not equate to losing independence or comfort.

The beauty of these devices lies in their ability to learn and adapt to our routines and preferences. A smart refrigerator can keep track of groceries and suggest shopping lists, while a smart oven can ensure that meals are cooked to perfection with minimal supervision. Gadgets like these are companions in the kitchen, helping us maintain a healthy and balanced diet, which becomes increasingly important as we age.

Beyond the kitchen, smart devices extend their reach to safety and security. Motion sensors and automated alerts provide peace of mind. The ability to monitor one's home remotely means that help is always within reach, and independence does not come at the cost of security.

The integration of smart technology into the home environment also fosters social connections. Video calling allows for face-to-face conversations with family and friends, bridging the gap that physical distance may create. It's a poignant reminder that the warmth of a smile or the comfort of a familiar face is only a few taps away.

Smart devices can also be used for personal growth and mental stimulation. They offer access to audiobooks, music, and podcasts, all of which can be enjoyed without fiddling with complex controls or small buttons. Keeping our minds active and learning new things is always important, no matter how old we are. Smart technology helps ensure that age doesn't stop us from continuing to learn and grow.

If you choose to integrate smart devices into your life, approach them with a sense of curiosity and patience. There is a learning curve, but it can be navigated with support and guidance. Many communities offer workshops and classes designed to help seniors become more comfortable with technology, and a growing number of resources are available online.

Aging with grace in the digital age is about balancing embracing new technologies and maintaining the essence of what makes life meaningful. Smart devices are tools, and when used thoughtfully, they can enhance our ability to live with meaning and connection.

E-Learning: Opportunities for Continued Education

The pursuit of knowledge keeps our lives full of fulfillment and activity. The digital age has opened up a treasure trove of opportunities for continued education that we might not have had before. Online learning, or E-learning, is a remarkable tool that empowers us to learn, grow, and thrive, regardless of our age.

Gone are the days when learning was confined to the four walls of a classroom or the pages of a textbook. Today, the world is our classroom, and the internet is our teacher, offering various courses, workshops, and seminars that cater to different interests and needs. Whether it's delving into the mysteries of ancient history, mastering a new language, or exploring the wonders of digital photography, e-learning platforms provide an accessible and flexible way to continue our education at our own pace and comfort.

For those of us who have witnessed the evolution of technology over the decades, the idea of online learning may initially seem intimidating. However, these platforms are designed with user-friendliness in mind. Many offer step-by-step tutorials and support systems to guide users through the process, ensuring that even those new to digital devices can easily navigate the learning environment.

E-learning is also about connecting with others who share our interests and passions. Virtual classrooms and forums create communities of learners, enabling us to engage in meaningful discussions, exchange ideas, and forge friendships that enrich our lives beyond the screen. This sense of community can be precious as we age, providing social interaction and intellectual stimulation that contribute to our well-being.

E-learning can be a source of empowerment and confidence. As we complete courses and gain new skills, we reinforce the understanding that age is not a barrier to learning. This can profoundly impact our self-esteem and perception of what it means to age with grace. It reminds us that our capacity for growth and adaptation is not diminished by the years we have lived but enhanced by the wisdom we have gained.

In embracing the opportunities for continued education that e-learning offers, we also set an example for future generations. We demonstrate that learning is a lifelong journey that enriches our lives and keeps us connected to the ever-evolving world around us.

Chapter Summary

- The internet provides a wealth of resources for all ages, acting as a bridge to the wider world and a source of endless knowledge.

- Thanks to the digital world, we can engage in lifelong learning through online courses and tutorials, exploring new subjects and keeping our minds sharp.
- The internet offers entertainment options like streaming services, e-books, and audiobooks, providing leisure and relaxation at home. However, the internet should be approached openly and cautiously, ensuring online safety through strong passwords and privacy awareness.
- Social media allows us to stay connected with loved ones, share experiences, and participate in global conversations.
- Smart devices can simplify daily tasks, enhancing safety, comfort, and social connections.

10

AGING IN PLACE: MAKING THE MOST OF YOUR HOME

A s we journey through the golden years of our lives, the familiar comfort of our homes becomes even more important to us. Within these walls, we have celebrated life's milestones, weathered tough times, and found peace in the quiet moments. Aging with grace means being able to adapt, and adapting our homes to meet our changing needs is a powerful way to look after ourselves.

Home modifications for safety and comfort affirm our desire to live life to its fullest, regardless of age. These modifications can range from simple additions to more extensive renovations, each to create an environment that is as safe as it is nurturing. Revisit the 'Art of Adaptation' chapter to learn how to modify your home to make your living spaces more manageable as you age.

These home modifications help prevent harm and enhance quality of life. They allow us to continue engaging with our passions, welcome family and friends, and live with autonomy.

Community Resources and Support Services

In old age, we may feel an increasing desire to remain in the familiar comfort of our homes. Aging in place is a choice many make, and it can be richly rewarding with suitable support systems in place. Beyond the physical modifications to our homes discussed earlier, a robust network of community resources and support services is pivotal in enabling this independence.

Community resources come in various forms, from local senior centers that offer socialization and recreational activities to meal delivery services that ensure proper nutrition when cooking becomes a challenge.

Transportation services, too, are an integral component of community support. They provide the means for individuals to maintain their autonomy to attend medical appointments, shop for groceries, or enjoy a change of scenery without the stress of driving. These services often include reduced fares or even door-to-door assistance for those with mobility issues.

Another invaluable resource is legal and financial counseling. As we age, navigating the complexities of estate planning, healthcare directives, and benefits can be overwhelming. Community-based programs often offer workshops or one-on-one counseling to help seniors confidently understand their rights and plan for the future.

Health and wellness programs tailored to the needs of older adults are also a cornerstone of community support. These may include exercise classes to maintain mobility and balance, health screenings, and educational seminars on managing chronic conditions.

Community resources and support services provide the practical assistance, emotional support, and sense of connection essential for a fulfilling and independent life at home. As we move forward, we will explore another type of support for those who wish to age in place: in-home care options.

In-Home Care: Options for Assistance

In-home care is a helpful source of help as we age, providing various services to match different needs and wants.

It is a compassionate way to balance the desire for autonomy with the help we might need, ensuring we stay safe, have company, and are well taken care of.

Personal care assistants, sometimes known as aides, can help us when we may not be as steady as they once were. They can assist with the daily rituals of living, like bathing, dressing, and grooming. For many, these tasks are intimate, and the presence of a gentle and respectful assistant can make all the difference in preserving dignity and comfort.

Healthcare at home is not limited to non-medical aid. Registered and licensed practical nurses are available for those requiring medical attention, from medication management to wound care. Their expertise is not just in the procedures they perform but in their ability to provide reassurance and understanding to those under their care.

Meal preparation services are another component of in-home care. Whether it's due to dietary restrictions or the simple challenge of cooking for one, having someone to prepare wholesome, balanced meals can nourish the body as much as the soul.

Mobility and the freedom it brings can sometimes be hindered as we age. Physical and occupational therapists can visit homes to provide exercises and strategies to maintain or improve mobility, ensuring that the home remains a place of freedom, not confinement.

Companionship, often overlooked, is as crucial as any medical service. Loneliness can become more common as we age, but companion services offer light through shared activities, conversation, and the simple, profound presence of another person. This companionship can range from a few hours a week to live-in support.

Choosing the right type of in-home care is a deeply personal decision that should be made with careful consideration of your needs, values, and financial circumstances. It is a collaborative process involving family, healthcare providers, and the individuals providing the care. Open communication about expectations, boundaries, and the evolving nature of your needs is essential to creating a supportive and adaptive environment.

Aging in place with the support of in-home care is about crafting a life stage not defined by limitations but by the possibilities that thoughtful assistance can provide. It is about continuing to write one's story at home, surrounded by the memories that echo through the halls and the new ones waiting to be made.

Downsizing: Simplifying Your Surroundings

Downsizing, or simplifying your surroundings, can be a natural step in aging gracefully. It's a proactive approach to making your home more manageable and suited to your changing lifestyle.

Downsizing is not just about letting go of possessions; it's about curating your space to improve your quality of life. It involves a thoughtful paring down of belongings that allows for easier maintenance and accessibility. This simplification can lead to a safer living environment, reducing the risk of accidents and ensuring daily tasks are less strenuous.

The first step in this journey is to assess your current living situation. Take stock of the items you use regularly and those that have gone untouched for years. It's helpful to categorize belongings into essentials, sentimental items, and things that can be donated or discarded. Remember, the goal is to retain what adds value to your life and supports your daily routine.

When it comes to sentimental items, try to find a balance. These pieces are tangible connections to our past but need not overwhelm our present. Consider keeping only a select few with the deepest meaning or evoke the fondest memories. You might also explore creative ways to preserve memories, such as converting photos into digital formats or crafting a memory quilt from old clothing.

It's also worth considering the future when downsizing. What modifications might you need to make to your home to accommodate potential mobility changes? Planning for these adjustments now can make transitions smoother down the line.

Downsizing can be emotional, and taking it one step at a time is okay. It's an opportunity to set the stage for a new chapter of life that prioritizes ease, safety, and joy. Remember, the space you create doesn't just house you; it should reflect and support who you are at this stage of life.

Family, friends, and professionals can offer support and guidance throughout the process. They can help you make decisions, assist with the physical aspects of downsizing, and provide emotional support as you navigate this change.

Downsizing can pave the way for a home that continues to be a source of comfort and where you can age with grace and dignity. It's about making room in your home and your life for new experiences, relationships, and the peace that comes with a simplified, harmonious environment.

The Emotional Aspects of Aging in Place

Our homes are treasure chests full of memories, painting the picture of our lives. Every room is filled with the sounds of past laughter, the quiet of old talks, and the marks of memorable moments. These memories become a big part of who we are as we age. Growing old in our home keeps us tied to these stories, giving us a comforting sense of ongoing life. The walls around us become part of who we are, offering a warm hug in a world that always seems to be moving and shifting.

The choice to age in place also has unique emotional challenges. The passage of time may alter our relationship with our home. Rooms once filled with the energy of a bustling family may now stand quieter, prompting feelings of loneliness or loss. Maintaining a household that once seemed effortless can become a source of stress or frustration as our physical abilities shift.

If you begin to experience these feelings, sit with them and understand that they are a natural response to the changes that aging brings. Recognizing the resilience and adaptability that come with age is just as important. We learn to find new rhythms and create new routines that honor our current selves while staying true to the essence of our home.

To manage the emotional complexities of aging in place, it is beneficial to cultivate a supportive community, whether it be through neighbors, friends, family, or local services. Social connections can transform the experience of aging in place from one of isolation to one of engagement and purpose. Inviting others into our space for a cup of tea, a shared meal, or simply a chat can breathe new life into our homes and our hearts.

Personalizing your living space to reflect your current lifestyle and passions can reinvigorate your emotional bond with your home. This could mean converting a child's old bedroom into a space for a new hobby or interest or redesigning a living area to host gatherings for book clubs or game nights. By doing so, you can create an environment that accommodates your physical needs and nourishes your emotional well-being.

Aging in place is a journey that is as much about the heart as the home. It is about creating a sanctuary that shelters our aging bodies and cradles our evolving spirits.

Chapter Summary

- Aging in place involves adapting homes to meet changing needs and enhancing safety, comfort, and independence.
- Home modifications can include better lighting, slip-resistant flooring, bathroom grab bars, and accessible kitchen designs.
- Community resources and support services provide socialization, meal delivery, transportation, legal and financial counseling, and health programs as we age.
- In-home care options range from personal care assistants to medical professionals, offering services like

meal preparation, mobility assistance, and companionship.
- Downsizing involves simplifying living spaces by decluttering and reorganizing to improve safety and manageability.
- The emotional aspects of aging in place include maintaining a connection to personal history and adapting to changes in the home environment.
- Cultivating a supportive community and personalizing living spaces can help combat loneliness and enhance emotional well-being.
- Aging in place is a holistic approach that considers physical, emotional, and social needs to create a comfortable and meaningful living environment.

CLOSING THOUGHTS AND REFLECTIONS

As we walk the path of life, we collect a mosaic of experiences, each teaching us a lesson that adds to the wisdom we carry forward. When we reflect on our life's journey, especially during our later years, we see all the things we've learned and the elegance with which we've moved through our days.

One of the most significant lessons is the art of resilience. Life challenges our strength and flexibility in its unpredictable ebb and flow. Aging with grace teaches us that resilience is not about avoiding the storm but learning to dance in the rain. It's about finding happiness amid sorrow, strength in vulnerability, and growth in adversity.

Another lesson is the importance of relationships. The value of deep, meaningful connections becomes ever more apparent as the years pass. These relationships—be they with family, friends, or community members—form the foundation of our support system. They offer love, laughter, and comfort, reminding us that we are not solitary travelers but part of a rich narrative of human connection.

We also learn the lesson of letting go. With age comes the understanding that not everything in life can be controlled. Letting go of past wrongs, unmet expectations, and roads not taken frees us to live more fully in the present. It allows us to forgive ourselves and others, release the weight of what we cannot change, and cherish the moments that bring light to our days.

The journey teaches us about the beauty of simplicity. As the clutter of earlier decades falls away, the simple pleasures come into sharper focus. A cup of tea in the quiet of the morning, the laughter of our family, the comfort of a well-loved book—these simple joys become the highlights of our days, reminding us that happiness often resides in the smallest moments.

Lastly, aging with grace imparts the wisdom of gratitude. Each year, we become more acutely aware of life's fragility and the gift each day presents. Gratitude becomes a daily practice, a way of seeing the world that enriches our experience and fills us with peace and contentment.

As we reflect on these lessons, we realize that aging is both a physical process but a spiritual and emotional journey. It is a time to harvest the wisdom sown throughout our lives, share it with others, and prepare ourselves for the next chapter with an open heart and a spirit of anticipation. The journey, with all its twists and turns, has brought us to a place of introspection and understanding—a place where we can look back with appreciation and look forward with hope.

The Gift of Memories: Cherishing the Past

Our memories are the vibrant colors that give richness and depth to our lives. They are the narrative of our journey, a collection of moments, both big and small, that have shaped who we are. To age with grace is to cherish these memories and hold them close as treasured keepsakes.

Memories are more than just recollections of past events; they are the legacy of our emotions and experiences. They are the laughter that echoed through the halls of a childhood home, the warmth of a loved one's embrace, and the bittersweet tears of a farewell that was not the end but a transition. In our later years, these memories become integral to our identity, the stories we share with younger generations, and the wisdom we impart.

Cherishing the past does not mean living in it but rather honoring it. It is about acknowledging the struggles we've overcome, the love we've given and received, and the knowledge we've gained. It is about recognizing that every challenge faced and every joy embraced has contributed to the strength and resilience that characterizes a life well-lived.

As we age, we may find that our memories begin to fade, like the soft edges of an old photograph. However, this does not diminish their value. Instead, it invites us to revisit them, speak about them, and write them down, ensuring that they continue to live on for those who will follow in our footsteps.

The gift of memories is also a reminder of our shared humanity. It connects us to others, creating a connection that is not solely our own but part of a larger, more intricate network. Our stories intertwine with those of our friends, family, and even strangers, creating a narrative that spans time and space.

In this reflective space, we find comfort and joy in the memories we've cultivated. We understand that while our physical abilities may wane, the mind's garden of memories remains fertile, ready to be tended and appreciated.

In the calmness of our later years, when the hustle of life slows to a gentler pace, we have the precious opportunity to sift through these memories and find peace in knowing that our lives have been a collection of meaningful moments.

Embracing the Present: The Power of Now

The true art of aging with grace can be found in embracing the present. The present is a canvas upon which the colors of every yesterday and the light of each tomorrow blend into the masterpiece of now.

Living in the present means accepting the symphony of life with all its ups and downs. It means sitting in the garden of existence, inhaling the fragrance of blooming flowers without lamenting yesterday's fallen petals or wishing for tomorrow's buds.

The present is also a sanctuary of acceptance. It is where age is not a sign of wear but a badge of honor, reflecting the resilience and the stories etched in the lines of a well-lived life. Here, in the power of now, there is no need for the facades of youth because the beauty of the present is in the authenticity of the self, the comfort of one's skin, and the peace that comes with self-acceptance.

The present is where we can cultivate happiness and engage with the world around us with curiosity and wonder. It is where we can share the wisdom gleaned from years of experience, laugh with the innocence of a child, and impart the warmth of our spirit to those whose lives we touch.

Looking Forward: Hope and Aspirations

As we add the last details to our story of growing old gracefully, we look ahead to a future filled with hope and aspirations. It's like looking at the soft glow of the morning sun, hinting at the beginning of a new adventure even as we finish the current one.

In a life full of rich experiences, each event is a unique thread—a lesson, a treasured moment. As we age, these threads become interwoven with wisdom, resilience, and a deeper appreciation of the beauty of life. Our aspirations aren't just idle hopes; they are beacons that guide us, illuminating the path ahead with purpose and new opportunities.

Hope encourages us to picture a future where our wisdom enables us to contribute in ways we never thought possible. It is the gentle hand on our back that propels us forward, reminding us that our presence, stories, and insights are valuable gifts to the world around us.

As we look forward, we aspire to embody the grace we have cultivated. We think about sharing our narratives with younger generations, not as a blueprint for living but to show how one can navigate the waters of existence. We aspire to be mentors, friends, and confidants, offering our experiences as a lantern in the night for those who may find themselves lost in the shadows of uncertainty.

We seek to embrace the joy of living and find beauty in the simplicity of a morning's sunrise or the laughter of a loved one. We continue growing, learning, and loving with the fullness of our beings, for it is in these pursuits that we can find life's truest pleasures.

In the quiet moments of reflection, we may find ourselves

yearning for a sense of peace and contentment. This is the ultimate aspiration: to reach a place within ourselves where the bustle of life is met with a calm that comes from knowing we have lived authentically, loved deeply, and left a legacy of kindness and compassion.

We move forward with the understanding that each day is a precious opportunity to add another stroke of beauty to the masterpiece of our lives.

Your Graceful Path Forward

Let's take a moment to reflect on what it means to have aged gracefully. Aging with grace involves a daily commitment to embracing the beauty of our years and the wisdom that comes with it. It is a path we build with patience, kindness, and a deep appreciation for the little moments that make up our lives.

To age with grace is to understand that every wrinkle is a story, every gray hair a badge of honor, and every shared laugh a treasure. It means accepting the past without regret, living in the present with exhilaration, and approaching the future without fear.

Remember that you are alone on this journey. You are part of a community that has also journeyed through the seasons of life, each person with their unique narrative. Together, we can support and uplift one another, sharing the joys and shouldering the burdens that come over time.

Remember also that grace is not a static state but a dynamic process. It requires adaptability, an open heart, and a willingness to learn and grow. It asks that we remain curious, engaged, and connected to the world around us, never losing sight of the wonder life offers at every age.

In embracing this path forward, we acknowledge that the fullness of life is not diminished by age but rather enriched by it. We carry within us the pieces of every person we have loved, every challenge we have overcome, and every moment of beauty we have witnessed. These pieces connect to form the magnificent artwork of our existence, which is ever-evolving and uniquely ours.

As you continue to fill your canvas, do so with the understanding that aging is not a process of losing yourself but a continuous discovery of who you are meant to be. May your days be filled with purpose, your heart with compassion, and your life with the grace that comes from knowing you have lived well, loved deeply and left a legacy of poise and strength.

In the quiet moments of reflection, may you look upon your life with gentle pride and a new-found gratitude for the journey. Through the culmination of our years, we can truly understand the depth of our resilience, the power of our connections, and the beauty of a life well-lived.

ABOUT THE AUTHOR

Hanna Bentsen is an expert in the art of mindful aging and intentional living. With a compassionate voice and a wealth of experience, her work revolutionizes the way we perceive aging and life's inevitable transitions and redefines the middle and later years as periods of growth and enrichment.

Her insightful explorations into Swedish Death Cleaning and the art of aging with grace challenge societal norms, encouraging readers to approach decluttering and aging with intention and dignity. Hanna's books empower readers to embrace the later stages of life with newfound purpose and vitality. They offer practical wisdom for decluttering life's physical and emotional spaces.

Hanna's love for Scandinavian culture, with its emphasis on simplicity and functionality, deeply influences her approach to a well-lived life.

www.ingramcontent.com/pod-product-compliance
Lightning Source LLC
Chambersburg PA
CBHW071718020426
42333CB00017B/2318